VEGAN COOKBOOK

FOR ATHLETES

- Bank PKO BP
- writer. com f

SCOTT NARDELLA

To Enza, my wife

Table of contents

INTRODUCTION	**11**
CHAPTER 1	**16**
VEGAN DIET FOR ATHLETES	**16**
TOP TIPS FOR HIGH-PERFORMANCE VEGETARIAN ATHLETES	17
BENEFITS OF A VEGAN DIET FOR ATHLETES	19
NUTRITION TIPS FOR VEGAN ATHLETES	23
NUTRITIONAL GUIDELINES FOR ATHLETES	28
SOME COMMON ATHLETE'S ISSUES	32
CHAPTER 2	**38**
VEGANISM AS A LIFESTYLE	**38**
VARIOUS TYPES OF VEGAN DIETS	39
VEGAN DIETS CAN HELP YOU LOSE WEIGHT	41
THE VEGAN DIETS, THE BLOOD SUGAR AND TYPE 2 DIABETES	42
THE VEGAN DIETS AND THE HEART HEALTH CONDITION.	43
OTHER HEALTH BENEFITS FOR PEOPLE ON VEGAN DIETS.	44
FOODS TO AVOID	45
FOODS TO EAT	46
RISKS OF VEGANISM AND HOW TO MINIMIZE THEM	48
SUPPLEMENTS TO CONSIDER	50
EATING VEGAN AT RESTAURANTS	52
HEALTHY VEGAN SNACKS	53
CHAPTER 3	**55**

19 MYTHS ON VEGANISM   55

1. Vegans Need Supplements   56
2. Veganism Is an Eating Disorder   57
3. Veganism is for Hippies and Hipsters   58
4. Veganism Is a Trend   59
4. Vegan Diet Is not Good for Children and Pregnant Women   60
5. Vegan Pet Diets Are Dangerous   61
6. Fishes and Animals do not Feel Pain   62
7. It is Impossible to be Vegan if You Live or Travel Abroad. Eating Out as a Vegan Is Impossible!   63
8. Soya (Soy) Is Destroying the Environment and the Rainforests   64
9. Vegans Only Eat Processed Foods   65
10. Veganism Is Impossible for Athletes, Your Workout Will Suffer   65
11. You Need Meat For Muscle Building   66
12. Tofu and Soy Contain Estrogen, which Lowers Testosterone and Gives You Cancer   67
13. Plantations Business Kills Many Animals   68
14. Vegan Diet Gives Less Energy   68
15. It Is Impossible to Be a Vegan Since Animal Products Are Everywhere   69
16. We Should Worry About Other Problems in the World, not About Animals   71
17. People With Food Allergies Can not Be Vegans   72
18. I Can not Be Vegan when My Family, Partner, or Roommate Is not   73
19. Being a Vegan Guarantees Weight Loss. Veganism Is Always Healthy   74

CHAPTER 4   75

PROTEIN: MYTHS AND FACTS FOR ATHLETES   75

1. The Need for Protein   76
2. The Amount of Protein Needed for an Athlete   77
3. Is the Vegan Diet Protein Deficient?   78
4. Is the Protein Gotten from Meat Better than the Protein Gotten Elsewhere?   79
5. Eating too Much / too Little Protein Causes Diseases   80

6. What to Do if Protein Deficient?   81

7. The Vegan Protein Sources   82

CHAPTER 5   **86**

NUTRITIONAL FACTS ABOUT VEGAN DIET   **86**

Macronutrients   87

Micronutrients   94

Muscle Gain Macros   101

Macro Meal Planning   102

Vegan Protein   103

High Protein Foods for Vegans   104

Vegan Protein Absorption   109

CHAPTER 6   **114**

VEGAN ATHLETES FOOD FOR WORKOUT   **114**

Vegan Grocery List   114

Pre Workout Vegan Meals   117

Post-Workout Vegan Meal   120

CHAPTER 7   **127**

A 4 WEEKS VEGAN MEAL PLAN   **127**

Week One   127

Week Two   132

Week Three   136

Week Four   140

Nutrition Guide and Sources of Nutrients   144

CHAPTER 8   **150**

HIGH PROTEIN VEGAN RECIPES FOR ATHLETES   **150**

Vegan Breakfast Recipes   **151**

Vegan Breakfast Sandwich   152

Vegan Crepes   154

Mango Craze Juice Blend   155

Strawberry Oatmeal Smoothie   156

Country Style Fried Potatoes   157

Kale and Banana Smoothie   158

Homemade Soy Yogurt   160

Pumpkin Pie Cake   162

Vegan Lunch Recipes   **164**

Crunchy Red Cabbage and Green Apple Sesame Slaw   165

Plate of mixed greens   166

Smoky Avocado and Jicama Salad   168

Mango, Kale, and Avocado Salad   169

Stewed Butternut Squash and Apple Soup   170

Curried Yellow Lentils With Avocado   172

Kale Salad With Apple and Creamy Curry Dressing.   173

Red Quinoa, Cantaloupe, and Arugula Salad   175

Hot Thai Salad   176

Carrot Avocado Bisque   177

Gluten-free Tortilla Pizza   178

Cashew Cheese   179

Vegan Dinner Recipes   **181**

Beans and Quinoa Salad   182

Zucchini Pasta, with Cherry Tomatoes, Basil, and Hemp Parmesan   184

Hemp Parmesan   185

Gluten-free White Bean and Summer Vegetable Pasta   185

Butternut Squash Curry   187

Zucchini Alfredo with Basil and Cherry Tomatoes   189

6

Vegan Dips and Dressings   **191**

Turmeric Tahini Dressing   192

Walnut Pesto   193

Balsamic Tahini Dressing   194

Rich Apricot Ginger Dressing   195

Fig and White Balsamic Vinaigrette   196

Vegan Snacks   **197**

Vegan Peanut Butter   198

Hemp Hummus   200

Peanut Butter And Jelly Snack Balls   201

Sweet Potato Hummus   202

Vegan Za'atar Crackers   203

Vegan Smoothies   **206**

Avocado Banana Nuts Smoothie   207

Banana Hemp Seed Smoothie   208

Mango Tahini Smoothie   209

Ingredients: 209

Cucumber Pear Smoothie   210

Smoothie Bowl with Mango and Coconut   211

Cashew Butter Smoothie with Banana, Berry, Dates, and Flax   212

INTRODUCTION

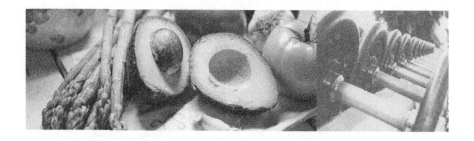

As an athlete, your diet is as important as your training session. Adequate planning makes it easy about dieting. Being on a vegan diet, especially for an athlete, will require planning meals for more days. The food requires a large number of nutrients and ingredients, consequently, the planning. To start with, the calories to be taken in is essential. If somebody wants to develop mass and build the body, they need to take in a more significant number of calories than the body usually requires. As a beginner athlete, you have to take in in any event 10 percent extra of what your body burns on an average day. If the calories are insufficient, it will not be easy to build your body to suit your desire.

Regardless of whether you are a sprinter, track athlete, field athlete, high jumper, swimmer, volleyballer, basketballer or a cyclist, you want to get progressively fit, with a vegan diet and great workout. As a rule, exercise, if done wrong, can be traced back to a wrong lifestyle: the absence of rest, stress, or inappropriate food (or just insufficient food).

Since protein is of particular significance for athletes, either male or female, and we decided to get rid of eating animals and animal products, plant-based protein is the obvious choice. Foods like Tempeh, Tofu, Quinoa, Brown Rice, and Seitan are wealthy in protein and will give the required amount to get progressively fit as an athlete. Quinoa is likewise important, as it is well known because it is a perfect source of protein. It is incredibly high in protein. What you have to know as an athlete is that you need to eat enough to get the ideal outcomes.

For most athletes who double as bodybuilders, there is an 'on-season' and an 'off-season.' Later, it is fitting to take in a high measure of calories and protein. As a vegan bodybuilder, it is sensible to add weight. The off-season represents the building stage. It is during the on-season that the accumulated fat and weight gets chopped down.

A Vegan athlete should not have any issue with this stage as plant-based meals are known for helping weight loss. Exercises during this period tend towards being light and retaining muscle mass. Feeding, as well, is centred on a similar goal as exercises. The main distinction is that calories are cut just as fat intake. The building stage and the cutting stage depend on the calories from the primary macronutrients in a vegan diet, which is protein, carbs, and fats. Building muscles and the body, largely, may not be agreeable in a DIY mode, so it is smarter to work with a dietitian or nutritionist. Two distinct people cannot intake a similar quantity of calories, or have their metabolisms working at the same rate, which implies, at last, the experience and guidance of an expert (nutritionist) would consistently stay substantial. Besides the fundamental macronutrients recorded above, it is fitting to eat a lot of fruits or fruit products, and minerals. They could come close by meals or fill in as the primary course as servings of mixed greens. It could be a tidbit based on your nutritionist's recommendation. Organic products are, for the most part, plentiful in nutrients and minerals. Nutrients, thus, are exceptionally gainful to the body. They go about as cancer prevention agents as well. A stable and healthy body is expected to remain fit and workout; in this manner, the presence of products of fruit and minerals is irreplaceable in a vegan diet.

To take advantage of a vegan diet as an athlete, you should avoid refined foods; however, much as could be expected, eating healthy and clean is the key. The motivation behind why prepared foods should not exist in your diet is that you might be deprived of the whole nutrient of what you are taking in. A few people feel the main thing they have to be careful about is the presence of animal protein, so they start to take snacks high in carbs. There is not a viable alternative for being on a raw diet as the outcomes are the best. Taking in a lot of liquids also is a piece of the way toward getting fit on a vegan diet. A vegan diet is a diet that is high in fiber, which implies deficient intake of liquids could bring about some symptoms, for example, an enlarged stomach or stomach problems. The most widely recognized and helpful juice that can work best is water. First of all, against the calories taken in. Taking at least 1milliliter per calorie is sufficient.

Besides eating well indeed, supplements can help to up everything. The explanation behind supplements is that diets would not give the whole nutrients required by wellness. Being on a tight eating routine leaves space for insufficiency, regardless of how 'complete' the diet might be. The danger of imperfection can drop by having a wide assortment of food to browse for on your diet menu. Supplements should be utilized to compensate for what is absent. Nutrients like Vitamin B12, Vitamin D, and Omega-3 may not be sufficient for vegan diets. Getting supplements could really help. The body does not effortlessly retain the type of Iron acquired from plant sources. Specialists exhort supplementing this with Vitamin C to help its absorption.

About working out, it is exceptionally safe to spend a brief period as a new vegan bodybuilder. Along these lines, you will not lose such an enormous amount as far as mass. Working out for a critical time frame would cause your body to depend more on protein to finish the workouts. The shorter your workout sessions, the more protein you have coming up, which likewise helps the development of mass at last. For snacks, you can generally nibble on products of fruit and minerals. Nuts furnish healthy fats that will help with enduring energy, particularly during workouts. Nuts are valuable as far as muscle gain. Taking all things together, bodybuilding on a vegan diet verges on precise standards, eat enough and eat consistently, get enough rest, do not prepare more than would generally be appropriate, and take in the correct macros. You are gaining the necessary muscle and weight after all these are not hard in any way.

CHAPTER 1

VEGAN DIET FOR

ATHLETES

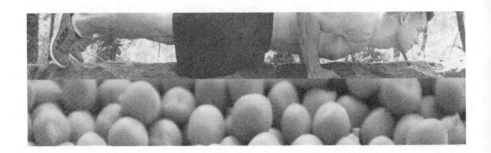

You can take the vegan diet to the extent you need it, some veggie lovers and vegan athletes incline toward crude and sans gluten diets, reporting importantly more significant energy gains.

You do not need to take it that far to see the benefits. There are contrasting degrees of health in plant-based diets, and includes a ton of delightful cooked foods that people following more customary diets would eat.

A vegan diet furnishes athletes with all the protein, complex starches, and different nutrients they have to get more grounded and quicker, without the conduit stopping cholesterol and saturated fats found in meat, eggs, and dairy items.

Vegans have lower rates of coronary illness, diabetes, heftiness, and many other kinds of disease than meat-eaters.

Top Tips for High-Performance Vegetarian Athletes

A reasonable, balanced veggie lover diet will give you the essential nutrients you need exceeding expectations. Here are a few things to recollect:

- Nutritionists prescribe that the vast majority of the calories athletes take in originate from complex starches. While refined carbohydrates like sugar and white bread should be avoided, complex carbs are essential for filling your muscles with energy in a continuous manner. Significant examples are whole wheat bread and pasta, grains, dark rice, quinoa, and products of fruit and minerals.

- Protein can be found plentiful in foods like beans, nuts, tofu, whole grains, veggie burgers, and Garden burger's meatless grill ribs, Boca's Chicken Nuggets, and other meat substitutes. Even though veggie lovers can without much of a stretch get a lot of protein through these foods, in case you're searching for a post-workout help, put some fruit products and minerals vegan protein supplement into a blender for a delicious smoothie, stir up a Vega drink, or snatch a delectable Clif Bar (counting as 20 grams of protein) from your neighbourhood store.

- A bit of fat in your diet is essential, and the fats in plant foods like avocados, vegetable and olive oils, nuts, and seeds will, in general, be a lot healthier than the supply route stopping up fats found in most animal products. Take a pass on pan-fried foods.

- Adding a multivitamin and a vitamin B12 supplement to your day-by-day diet is a smart thought for all athletes.

- Any coach will tell you that the more calories you burn, the more fuel you need. Vegan foods will, in general, be nutrient, yet they are, to some degree, less caloric than animal products. So eat many of your preferred plant-based dishes.

Benefits of a Vegan Diet for Athletes

A nutritious diet is key to the preparation and performance of an athlete. The type of diet they regularly have is the extra sparkle they have to perform at a specific rate and have a preferred position over different adversaries. Plant-based diets have gotten very famous in recent years. Diet has become an essential part of preparing and into what nutrition is a healthier decision for athletes is getting forced rapidly. A vegan diet carries a lot to an athlete's preparation and performance. Look at eight benefits that athletes can pick up by going vegan.

Athletic Performance Improvement

Many sports people and athletes have turned towards a vegan diet for better wellness and performance. While there are recommendations that a vegan diet might not have as much protein as in a non-vegan one, there are studies that show that vegans have a superior and improved physical wellness level than those taking a non-vegan diet. Other than proteins, it is essential to have a decent intake of different nutrients that help during the recuperation period. Therefore, numerous athletes are following a proper fat, nutrient, and mineral-rich vegan diet that improves their performance in sports.

Increase in Nutrients and Vitamins

Athletes have different nutritional needs to keep up a high standard. A vegan diet improves nutritional intake, particularly that of vitamins. Vitamins are essential for athletes. Acute physical exercise may bring about marginally suppressed safe capacity by expanding the job of healthy performer cells and neutrophils. It is realized that this move in the immune system raises the defenselessness to bacterial contaminations and undermines practice. Athletes need to prevent illness, and it has been demonstrated that the people who take a vegan or high in plant foods diet seem to become ill less frequently, conceivably in light of the safe properties of these foods.

Inflammation Decrease

Meat-eating and elevated cholesterol levels escalate exhaustion, which can prompt uneasiness and prevent athletic performance and recuperation. Studies show that a vegan diet has an anti-inflammatory impact. A diet based on vegetables, low in saturated fat, and liberated from cholesterol, improves the consistency or thickness of the blood. It permits the muscles to get more oxygen, which enhances performance in sports.

Better Mood

Vegans seem to be more joyful than their meat-eating counterparts might. It was found that vegans had lower scores on depression tests and temperament profiles when compared with meat-eaters. It is said that there is a component of freshness to most plant-based dishes, which helps to cleanse our brains and keep our musings positive.

Improved Cardiovascular Health

The more positive cardiovascular system helps with guaranteeing you can run quicker, hop higher, and train more earnestly all the time with quick recuperation periods between workouts. Since the plant-based diet is low in cholesterol and saturated fat, you can undoubtedly count on keeping up great cardiovascular health. If you have a cardiovascular system as fit as a fiddle, breathing, stamina, and in any event, remaining active all through your workouts and matches will be easier.

Physical Maintenance

Since plant-based diets are not loaded up with saturated fats, the physical maintenance you have to do as an athlete is genuinely easy to follow. Regardless of whether you are riding a bike and staying lean, or you need a sturdy and conditioned physical maintenance to karate fight, plant-based food will help you. A vegan diet consisting of a lot of grains, vegetables, natural products, and veggies is the base of any diet that advances health long haul.

Increased Energy

For our bodies, animal products are complex and hard to process and can prompt tiredness and exhaustion. Plants are high in nutrients, low in fat, and give you more calories. It has been proved that the wealth of starches improves quality and effectiveness for athletes, and whole grains, berries, and vegetables are the sugars to go for in a vegan diet.

Quicker Recovery

A vegan's recovery time might be shorter, and vegans are less inclined to injuries. Since vegan diets concentrated on whole food that includes numerous cancer prevention agents, they fight aggravation and stress frequently. Also, meat contains arachidonic acid, a highly inflammatory unsaturated fat, just as cortisol and c-responsive protein, which hinders recovery. A few athletes credit their diets concentrated on plants to expanded stamina and, in actuality, improved performance in their sports.

Going vegan can benefit numerous athletes. Diet is as important as training for the athletes, and a vegan diet can do a great deal of good to the athletes.

Nutrition Tips for Vegan Athletes

Below, this book will cover the nutritional basics for vegan athletes and all other dynamic people. From hydration to calming foods and getting enough protein, this should help you fill your diet with sustaining foods that will help fuel the dynamic way of life you love.

Hydration

The need of staying hydrated applies to anybody, yet it is so important I thought it has to be mentioned anyway. Your body cannot perform to its maximum capacity in case you are dehydrated.

Lack of hydration can cause:

- Fatigue

- Headaches

- Brain haze

- cramping

- decreasing performance

In addition, all these can themselves influence our health in different ways.

Stay Hydrated All Day

Make sure to drink enough water during your workouts as well as for the day too. Hydration is not something we can make up later, so it is imperative to hydrate reliably. I would suggest putting liquids into a water bottle you love and bring it with you wherever you go. When I work at home, I usually keep a 1 L bottle close to me consistently and try to finish three of them a day. When I am out on the town, I continually carry a water bottle with me.

If you have water with you, you will drink it!

Start Your Day with Water

Before you eat or drink whatever else in the first part of the day, hydrate. Drinking a good glass of water before anything else truly helps kick off the beginning of my day and improves energy. I go with a huge glass of water with lemon first thing each morning. You can likewise do a touch of lime or apple vinegar or lemon if you prefer. A pinch of sea salt can help with re-hydrating as it contains trace minerals.

Take Sports Drinks

In case you are practising intensely for more than 60 minutes-an hour and a half, consider an electrolyte drink, for example, coconut water, to recharge electrolytes lost through sweat. Coconut water is a good option in contrast to high-sugar sports drinks. You can likewise make your healthy sports drink by including some 100% natural juice and a touch of sea salt to your water bottle.

Consider Taking Supplements

Supplementation is not required however, it can be considered notwithstanding a whole food vegan diet. In case you are on a careful spending budget, do not stress over supplements, as supplements are only the tip of the iceberg of a different, nutrient whole food plant-based diet.

In case you have not previously failed with food quality, rest, hydration, and workout balance, there is no compelling reason to squander your cash on supplements. In case you are reliably eating clean, getting enough rest, hydrating reliably, and utilizing strategies to lessen pressure, at that point, you should think about using a few supplements. Yet, the difference they are going to make is unimportant.

Actual supplementation will rely upon your diet, your goals, and your activity level, so do some exploration and think about consulting with a nutritionist or RD on the off chance that you need some assistance.

Food First

Preferably, we'd take in every one of these vitamins and minerals through the foods we eat so make sure to include in your diet a lot of green leaves vegetables, beans, and almonds for calcium, pumpkin seeds, kale, nutty spread, molasses and apricots for Iron, and flax, chia and hemp seeds for essential fats.

The recommendations beneath are just supplements to consider, and I suggest doing your studies concerning what may be useful for you. Nothing is as incredible in a general food plant-based diet, so start there and afterwards think about supplements to fill in the holes.

The Only Essential Supplement B12

The main nutrient you have to supplement is Vitamin B12, which is very cheap. Search for a sublingual B12 splash that gives 500-1000 mcg of B12 and take that 2-3 times each week notwithstanding B12 supplemented foods, or every day in case you are not utilizing any supplemented foods. B12 strengthened foods include yeast, oats, and vegetable milk.

Other Supplements you can consider

- Omega-3 with DHA and EPA

- Creatine

- Vitamin D3

- Protein Powder

- Magnesium

Nutritional Guidelines for Athletes

Athletic men and women need more protein than other healthy people do. Frequently when animal products are wiped out from the diet, so it is a massive part of the protein. Without sufficient dietary protein, the sugar taken in will enter the circulation system quicker, causing insulin levels to rise rapidly (spike), and afterwards, a brief timeframe later decay (crash). With protein added to every meal, a "sugar crash" will not happen. Protein will supplement the starch, permitting it to enter the circulation system at a consistent rate, hence deferring the beginning of craving and supporting energy levels.

Protein, an important piece of an athlete's diet, is utilized in the rebuilding procedure of muscle tissue stressed by training. During aerobic exercise at a low pulse (60-70% of highest), fat is the body's essential fuel source (90%) with protein second (10%). Since Ironman and other intense exercise requires the body to be proficient at utilizing fat as fuel, long rides right now are necessary. A six-hour-ride, for instance, would burn only protein as fuel for 36 minutes.

If the dietary protein needs are not met for an athlete, muscle tissue will be catabolized; thus, the quality will decrease. A 4:1 starch to protein proportion appears to yield the best muscle glycogen recuperation results. The modest quantity of protein (25%) joined with a high glycemic starch (sugar) has appeared to improve recuperation over the ordinary "sugar only" approach. Supplemented soy drinks are a good supplier of this proportion.

Once animal products are disposed of, so is an enormous bit of the fat. The dairy business estimates fat as the level of volume, not as a level of calories. For instance, 2% milk is, in actuality, 33.5% fat. Eliminating all excess out of the diet is not the goal, albeit saturated fat should be limited for ideal performance. A low-fat diet is OK for a low to reasonably dynamic individual. Nevertheless, an exceptionally dynamic individual, particularly an athlete who follows a plant-based diet, will profit by adding high quality fats to his/her meals.

Likewise, with protein, fat helps with easing back the rate at which the sugar enters the circulation system, in this manner, giving supported, predictable energy. Dietary fat likewise helps the absorption of fat-solvent nutrients; for example, vitamin E. Vitamin E is a fantastic cancer prevention agent that will help stimulate the recuperation procedure. Cold-pressed oils, for example, flax and hemp, are incredibly essential to the vegan athlete. Both flax and hemp oils contain omega-3 unsaturated fats, and, above all, have anti inflammatory properties. These oils unfathomably speed the recuperation and fix of delicate tissue harm, the cost of every day preparing.

During times of level one (60-70% of most extreme pulse) aerobic exercise in the fat-burning zone (likewise known as metabolism preparing), the athlete should take in a mix of starch and protein.

Take in protein and high quality fat as a feature of every meal and bite.

Tip: If you make bread, biscuits, or any baked product, eliminate a portion of the flour and supplant it with soy protein powder, hemp flour, or bean flour. Use the hemp seed oil as a base for the plate of mixed greens dressing or to blend in with a soy drink to make it creamier. Use hemp seed oil on grain and in heating.

Excellent quality protein sources:

- Hemp seed nut and flour

- Tofu

- Beans (kidney, dark, garbanzo, soy, adzuki)

- Legumes

- Soy protein powder

- Unsweetened soy drink

Great quality fat sources:

- Extra virgin olive oil

- Flaxseed oil

- Hemp seed oil

- Avocado

- Non-broiled nuts and seeds

Some Common Athlete's Issues

Muscle cramps or contractions

Low sodium level: Lack of dietary sodium joined with normal sweating will drain sodium accumulation. Athletes who have embraced a plant-based diet are inclined to reduce sodium levels, frequently bringing about muscle cramps and contractions. Dairy items specifically contain elevated levels of sodium. Additionally, salami, pepperoni, baloney, and most complex prepared meats contain exceptionally elevated levels of sodium. Most plant sources have little sodium except for specific seaweeds. Inactive people, vegan or not, should not overlook this anyway.

During periods of intense training, delivering a high sweat rate, the vegan athlete will profit by salting his/her food. By adding sea salt to regularly eaten foods, the athlete will see that muscle stiffness dies down and suppleness returns. Because of excessive sweating, delivered by dashing in a hot domain, the athlete may require sodium tablets. Paving the way to a long race, for example, Ironman, the athlete must consider sufficient salt intake that will bring about lower reliance on race day. Salt accumulation will be preserved. A healthy, dynamic individual will not experience an ascent in circulatory pressure with the expansion of dietary sodium.

Low calcium level: The Low calcium levels in vegan athletes are, for the most part, caused by a mix of the absence of dietary calcium and hard preparation. Calcium is utilized during muscle withdrawals, causing numerous endurance athletes, vegan or not, to have diminished accumulation. For instance, an athlete who cycles for 5 hours at the standard rhythm of 90 revolutions for every moment will perform 54,000 muscle compressions. The withdrawals are from a blend of the three most significant muscles in the body (gluteus maximus, quadriceps, and hamstrings), a noteworthy draw on the body's calcium saves.

During intense preparation, a vegan athlete would profit from adding sea salt to at any rate one meal or nibble for every day. The week before a long race in a warm atmosphere, the athlete would profit by taking in sea salt at every meal.

An athlete who takes in calcium-rich foods at every meal will gain by creating supple, flexible muscles.

Tip: Add non-simmered sesame seeds to grain, servings of mixed greens, and whatever else you can consider. Sesame seeds are exceptionally high in calcium with 1-cup (250 ml) yielding 2900 mg of calcium. In correlation, 1 cup (250 ml) of dairy animals' milk contains 300 mg of calcium. It is a lot simpler to down some milk than some sesame seeds. However, once you remember them as a staple for your diet, they get in it rapidly.

To increase the absorption of calcium from sesame seeds, pound them in a coffee grinder. I suggest granulating a blend of sesame seeds and flax seeds and saving them in the ice chest for convenient, day-by-day use.

Calcium-rich foods include:

- Almonds

- Beans

- Dark, green leaves vegetables (spinach, kale)

- Sesame seeds

- Sunflower seeds

Low energy level

Reduced resilience to oxygen-consuming exercise; conceivable sickliness: When red meat is dispensed with from a functioning individual's diet, the long haul impact is frequently a decrease in red platelets regularly prompting iron deficiency. Vegan or not, athletes customarily experience issues keeping up acceptable iron levels for ideal performance. Support of iron accumulation turns out to be progressively troublesome during times of substantial preparation. Likewise, with sodium and calcium, Iron is lost in sweat, during warm weather, preparing largely a draw on iron accumulation. In contrast to sodium, iron levels can take as long as a half year to turn out to be perilously exhausted. Regularly not understanding this, the athlete will think about how performance has declined with no adjustment in diet or movement level. Since iron levels set aside impressive effort to be decreased, rebuilding takes equivalent time. A six-month-rebuilding stage would best be avoided. Iron is likewise lost because of compression hemolysis (squashed platelets because of extraordinary muscle withdrawals).

The more dynamic the individual, the more the dietary Iron is required. Steady effect action, for example, running, decreases iron levels all the more drastically because of a progressively strenuous type of hemolysis. With each foot strike, a limited quantity of blood is discharged from the harmed vessels. In time, this will cause iron deficiency if the athlete does not take care of diet.

Iron levels will consistently be uncovered and never permitted to get exhausted. Iron-rich foods are ideally consumed every day with vitamin C to help the absorption. If the running mileage is greater than 50 miles (80km), an iron supplement is suggested. Likewise, if preparing happens in a warm atmosphere (excessive sweating) all year, or preparing consistently surpasses 15 hours of the week, an iron supplement is suggested too.

Iron-rich foods:

- Fortified grain

- Split pea soup

- Cookies or other prepared foods made with molasses (likewise high in calcium)

- Dried peas and beans (kidney, lima, lentils)

- Bran

- Blackstrap molasses

- Soybean nuts

- Prune juice, raisins

- Enriched rice

- Peanut butter

- Apricots

- Green beans

- Walnuts, cashews, almonds

In case that a vegan diet is something you might want to attempt, ensure you go about it the correct way. On the chance that you have tried and failed previously, it is probably not entirely on you, you may just not have had all the info you needed.

CHAPTER 2

VEGANISM AS A LIFESTYLE

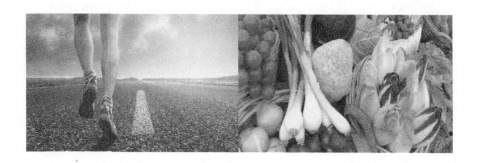

Veganism is known as a lifestyle that endeavours to reject all types of animal exploitation and killing, regardless of whether for food, garments, or any other reason.

Hence, the vegan diet is free from any animal product, including meat, eggs, and dairy.

People decide to follow a vegan diet for many different reasons.

These typically go from morals to environmental concerns, yet they can likewise come from a longing to improve health.

Various Types of Vegan Diets

There are various kinds of vegan diets. The best-known include:

- **The Whole-food vegan diet:** This is the diet that is based on a wide assortment of whole plant foods, for example, natural products, vegetables, whole grains, vegetables, nuts, and seeds.

- **The Raw-food vegan diet:** A vegan diet based on crude natural products, vegetables, nuts, seeds, or plant foods cooked at temperatures underneath 118°F (48°C).

- **The 80/10/10 diet**: This 80/10/10 diet method is a raw food vegan diet based on restriction of fat-rich plants, for example, nuts and avocados, and that depends predominantly on crude leafy foods greens. Additionally, alluded to as the low fat, crude food vegan diet, or fruitarian diet.

- **The starch arrangement:** A low fat, high-carb vegan diet like the 80/10/10 yet that centres around cooked starches like potatoes, rice, and corn rather than an organic product.

- **Raw Until 4:** A low-fat vegan diet inspired by the 80/10/10 and starch arrangement. Crude foods are eaten until 4 p.m., with the choice of a prepared plant-based meal for dinner.

- **The flourish diet:** The flourish diet is a crude food vegan diet. Adherents eat plant-based, whole foods that are crude or, eventually, cooked at low temperatures.

- **Junk-food vegan diet**: A vegan diet based less on whole plant foods that depend intensely on mock meats and cheeses, fries, vegan desserts, and other vigorously prepared vegan foods.

Although a few varieties of the vegan diet exist, and there are a few different ways to follow one, most research rarely separates between various kinds of vegan diets.

Hence, the data on this book refers to vegan diets in general, unless otherwise indicated.

Vegan Diets Can Help You Lose Weight

Vegans will, in general, be more slender and have a lower Body Mass Index (BMI) than non-vegans

This may explain why an expanding number of people go to vegan diets as an approach to lose excess weight.

Some portion of the weight-related benefits vegans experience might be clarified by factors other than diet. These may include a healthier way of life decisions, for example, physical action, and other health-related practices.

Vegan diets showed to be more successful for weight loss than the diets they have been compared with.

Strangely enough, the weight-loss advantage continues in any event, when all food-based diets are utilized as control diets.

Additionally, scientists report that people on vegan diets lose more weight than those following calorie-limited diets, in any event, when they are permitted to eat until they feel full.

The common inclination to eat fewer calories on a vegan diet might be brought about by a higher dietary fiber intake, which can make you feel fuller.

Vegan diets appear to be successful at helping people normally decrease the measure of calories they eat, bringing about weight loss.

The Vegan Diets, the Blood Sugar and Type 2 Diabetes

Embracing the vegan diet may help hold your glucose within proper limits and type two diabetes under control.

A few investigations show that vegans profit by lower glucose levels, higher insulin effectiveness, and go up to a 78% lower danger of acquiring type 2 diabetes than non-vegans.

Moreover, vegan diets purportedly lower glucose levels in people with diabetes up to 2.4 occasions more than diets prescribed by the ADA, AHA, and NCEP.

Some portion of the better results could be explained by the higher fiber consumption, which may dull the glucose reaction. A vegan diet's weight loss impacts may additionally add to the capacity to bring down glucose levels.

Vegan diets appear to be especially effective at improving markers of glucose control. They may likewise bring down the danger of creating type 2 diabetes.

The Vegan Diets and The Heart Health condition.

A vegan diet helps to keep the heart-healthy.

Vegans have up to a 75% lower risk of growing hypertension and a 42% lower risk of dying from coronary illness.

Randomized controlled research — the best quality level in inquiring — add to the proof. Vegan diets are considerably more effective at diminishing glucose, LDL, and all-out cholesterol than other diets they are compared with.

These impacts could be particularly valuable since diminishing circulatory pressure, cholesterol, and glucose may lessen coronary illness hazard by up to 46%.

Vegan diets may improve heart health. Nonetheless, increasingly top-notch contemplates are required before solid ends can be drawn.

Other Health Benefits For People on Vegan Diets.

Vegan diets are related to a variety of other health benefits, including benefits for:

- **Cancer chance:** Vegans may profit by a 15% lower danger of developing or passing on from cancer.

- **Arthritis:** Vegan diets appear to be especially effective at decreasing side effects of joint pain, for example, torment, and morning pain.

- **Kidney function:** The diabetics patients who substitute meat with plant protein may lessen their danger of poor kidney work.

- **Alzheimer's disease**: Observational investigations show that parts of the vegan diet may help diminish the danger of developing Alzheimer's disease.

Overall, remember that a large portion of the investigations supporting these benefits are observational. This makes it hard to decide if the vegan diet legitimately caused the benefits.

Randomized double-blind controlled researches are required before solid ends can be made.

Foods to Avoid

Vegans avoid eating any animal foods, just as any foods containing fixings obtained from animals.

These include:

- Meat and poultry: Beef, sheep, pork, veal, horse, organ meat, wild meat, chicken, turkey, goose, duck, quail, and so on.

- Fish and seafood: All types of fish, anchovies, shrimp, squid, scallops, calamari, mussels, crab, lobster, and so forth.

- Dairy: Milk, yoghurt, cheddar, spread, cream, dessert, and so on.

- Eggs: From chickens, quails, ostriches, fish, and so on.

- Bee items: Honey, honeybee dust, royal jelly, and so on.

- Animal-based fixings: whey, casein, lactose, egg white egg whites, gelatin, cochineal or carmine, isinglass, shellac, L-cysteine, animal inferred vitamin D3, and fish-determined omega-3 unsaturated fats.

Foods to Eat

Health-cognizant vegans substitute animal products with plant-based substitutions, for example:

- Tofu, seitan, and tempeh: These give a flexible protein-rich option instead of meat, fish, poultry, and eggs in numerous recipes.

- Legumes: Examples of foods like, beans, lentils, and peas, are superb sources of numerous nutrients and helpful plant mixes. Growing, maturing, and proper cooking can build nutrient absorption.

- Nuts and nut spread: Especially unroasted assortments, which are good sources of iron, fiber, magnesium, zinc, selenium, and vitamin E.

- Seeds: Especially chia, and flaxseeds, which contain a decent measure of protein and gainful omega-3 unsaturated fats.

- Calcium-sustained plant milk and yoghurt: These help vegans with accomplishing their suggested dietary calcium intakes. Choose assortments additionally invigorated with vitamins B12 and D at whatever point conceivable.

- Algae: Spirulina and chlorella are acceptable sources of complete protein. Different assortments are great sources of iodine.

- Nutritional yeast: This is a simple method to expand the protein substance of vegan dishes and include an intriguing gooey flavour. Pick vitamin B12-strengthened assortments at whatever point conceivable.

- Whole grains, oats, and pseudocereals: These are a great source of complex carbs, fiber, iron, B-nutrients, and a few minerals. Spelt, teff, amaranth, and quinoa are particularly high-protein choices.

- Sprouted and aged plant foods: Ezekiel bread, tempeh, miso, natto, sauerkraut, pickles, kimchi, and fermented tea regularly contain probiotics and vitamin K2. Growing and ageing can likewise help improve mineral absorption.

- Fruits and veggies: Both are great foods to build your vitamin intake. green leaves vegetables, for instance, bok choy, spinach, kale, watercress, and mustard greens, are especially high in iron and calcium.

Risks of Veganism and How to Minimize Them

You should prefer an all-around planned diet that cuts off points prepared foods and replaces them with nutrient-rich ones. This is rather important for everybody, not just vegans.

Overall, some vegan diets followers are especially in danger of certain nutrients lacking.

Truth be told, studies show that vegans are at a greater danger of having deficient blood levels of vitamin B12, vitamin D, long-chain omega-3s, iodine, iron, calcium, and zinc.

Not getting enough of these nutrients is troubling for everybody, except it might represent a specific hazard to those with expanded necessities, for example, kids or pregnant or breastfeeding women.

Your hereditary genetics and intestinal bacterial flora may likewise affect your capacity to determine the nutrients you need from a vegan diet.

Invigorated foods, particularly those with calcium, vitamin D, and vitamin B12 should likewise show up on your plate.

Besides, vegans needing to improve their absorption of iron and zinc should take a stab at maturing, growing, and cooking foods.

Likewise, the utilization of iron cast pots, avoiding tea or espresso with meals, and mixing iron-rich foods with a source of vitamin C can additionally help iron absorption.

In addition, the use of kelp or iodized salt to the diet can help vegans reach their suggested day-by-day intake of iodine.

Finally, omega-3 containing foods, particularly those high in alpha-linolenic acid (ALA), can enable the body to deliver longer-chain omega-3s, for example, eicosapentaenoic acid (EPA) and docosahexaenoic acid (DHA).

Foods high in ALA include chia, hemp, flaxseeds, pecans, and soybeans. Notwithstanding, there is a discussion with respect to whether this transformation is sufficiently proficient at addressing everyday issues.

In this manner, a day-by-day intake of 200–300 mg of EPA and DHA from a green growth oil supplement might be a more secure approach to prevent low levels.

Vegans might be at danger of certain nutrient shortages. A very well planned vegan diet that includes nutrient-rich whole and braced foods can help give sufficient nutrient levels.

Supplements to Consider

Some vegan may think that it is hard to eat enough of nutrient-rich or invigorated foods above to meet their everyday routines

Right now, the following supplements can be especially gainful:

- Vitamin B12: Vitamin B12 in cyanocobalamin structure is the most examined and appears to function admirably for a great many people.

- The Vitamin D: Option for D2 or vegan D3 structures, for example, those fabricated by Nordic Naturals or Viridian.

- EPA and DHA: Sourced from green growth oil.

- Iron: Should just be supplemented because of a recorded insufficiency. Ingesting an excessive amount of iron from supplements can cause health inconveniences and prevent the absorption of different nutrients.

- Iodine: Take a supplement or include 1/2 tsp of iodized salt to your diet day by day.

- Calcium: Calcium is best retained when taken in doses of 500 mg or less at once. Taking calcium simultaneously as iron or zinc supplements may decrease their absorption.

- Zinc: Taken in the zinc gluconate or the zinc citrate structures. Not to be taken simultaneously as calcium supplements.

Vegans unable to meet their prescribed nutrient intakes through foods or braced items alone should think about taking supplements.

Eating Vegan at Restaurants

Feasting out as a vegan can be testing.

One approach to diminish pressure is to get informed on vegan-accommodating eateries by utilizing sites, for example, happy cow or Veggie. Applications like VeganXpress and Vegman may likewise be useful.

When eating in a non-vegan restaurant, take a stab at checking the menu online in advance to perceive what vegan alternatives they may have for you.

Occasionally, calling early permits the chef to prepare something particularly for you. This grants you to show up at the place, sure that you will have something ideally more fascinating than a side plate of mixed greens.

When picking an eatery on the fly, make a point to get some information about their vegan choices when you step in, preferably before being seated.

If all else fails, settle on ethnic eateries. They will, in general, have dishes that are normally vegan accommodating or can be handily adjusted to turn out to be so. Mexican, Thai,

Middle-Eastern, Ethiopian, and Indian eateries will, in general, be great choices.

Once in the eatery, take a stab at distinguishing the veggie lover alternatives on the menu and asking whether the dairy or eggs can be removed to accommodate the dish to make it vegan.

Another simple tip is to arrange a few vegan starters or side dishes to make up a meal.

Healthy Vegan Snacks

Snacks are a great method to stay healthy and keep hunger under control between meals.

Some intriguing, versatile vegan alternatives include:

- Fresh, natural product with a spot of nut spread

- Hummus and vegetables

- Nutritional yeast sprinkled on popcorn.

- Roasted chickpeas

- Nut and natural product bars

- Trail blend

- Chia pudding

- Homemade biscuits

- Whole-wheat pita with salsa and guacamole

- Cereal with plant milk

- Edamame

- Whole-grain wafers and cashew nut spread

- A plant-milk latte or cappuccino

- Dried seaweed snacks

At whatever point planning a vegan snack, try to opt on fiber-and-protein-rich alternatives, which can help keep craving under control.

CHAPTER 3

19 MYTHS ON VEGANISM

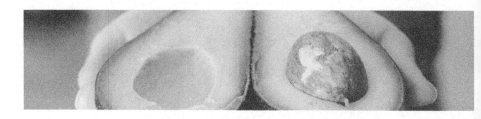

Regardless of whether actually intended or as only a joke, veganism has been the subject of a lot of deception.

For your inquisitive peruse, we are here to clear up many of these gossipy tidbits and myths.

1. Vegans Need Supplements

On the off chance that only vegans need supplements, at that point, how would you explain the bodybuilders, athletes, and athletes who do not follow a similar diet and still load up on supplements?

It is essential to comprehend what the term supplements really imply. Supplements supplement your diet. This implies they can be valuable to fill in the nutritional holes to help you with accomplishing your goals. Supplements do not (and ought not) supplant whole foods.

Truly, when following a vegan diet, there is a worry about getting enough Vitamin B12, Iron, Calcium, and Vitamin D. Saying this does not imply that it is difficult to get these nutrients on a vegan diet by means of whole foods. Alternatively, maybe, it is to a greater level an "in the event that something goes wrong" for what it's worth with most dietary supplements.

For instance, you need not bother with Vitamin D supplements throughout the winter; however, most specialists will prescribe this supplement because of the absence of common daylight during the colder months.

2. *Veganism Is an Eating Disorder*

An eating issue is described as a mental issue.

That implies there is a strange arrangement of conduct eating designs originating from various potential mental components.

At the end of the day, an eating issue is an ailment of the brain that is not willful and requires proficient help to cure.

Veganism, then again, is a cognizant decision made by an individual.

People who follow a vegan diet and a vegan lifestyle are not experiencing a mental illness.

This kind of vegan myth is offensive to both vegans and those really experiencing a devastating eating issue.

3. Veganism is for Hippies and Hipsters

This myth on veganism is based on unadulterated obliviousness.

Have you thought about the fact that there are dietary and strict practices over the world that advances a vegan way of life and diet?

Veganism and vegetarianism are certifiably not an advanced development of white radicals. It has been a lifestyle since the hour of our progenitors. To state that veganism is just for white flower children in the new age, is like saying that only people from Thailand are Buddhist or just Indians practice yoga.

It is a big world out there, and, in all honesty, people from all foundations follow a vegan diet and a vegan lifestyle.

4. Veganism Is a Trend

You can rapidly dispose of this myth just by understanding what the term trend implies.

A trend implies something that increases a fantastic measure of prominence for a short measure of time and afterwards observes a quick decrease in adherents. For instance, a year ago's design tendencies are a trend. They will be supplanted with a different line of style this year.

Veganism is a long way from a trend, or it is the longest trend to have happened. Studies and research can demonstrate that the cognizant decision to refrain from animal products goes back to a large number of years.

4. Vegan Diet Is not Good for Children and Pregnant Women

Naturally, people have worries about giving enough essential nutrients to developing kids and pregnant women. In any case, the possibility that a vegan diet some way or another comes up short on those nutrients is bogus.

The greatest determiner of malnutrition for youngsters and pregnant women is anything but a particular diet decision; rather, the financial status of the person.

If you cannot stand to purchase food, it does not make a difference in which diet you are attempting to follow.

Studies do make it a point to recommend supplements for a vegan diet, as we tended to above.

In any case, they likewise affirm that as long as vegans and veggie lovers follow the rules proposed in the Recommended Daily Allowance of the CDC, they will not need to stress over malnutrition.

Youngsters and pregnant women must follow a solid and steady vegan diet. This implies setting aside the effort to plan macronutrients, calories, and meals viably.

5. Vegan Pet Diets Are Dangerous

The next individual from the family that you might be worried about putting on a vegan diet is your pet. Since they are animals, it is anything but difficult to expect that they eat different animals. This is not valid.

While many pet proprietors can verify that it is so hard to keep a feline on a vegan diet, hound proprietors discover it shockingly simple. A vegan diet for a canine is just risky when the pooch's nutritional needs are not met. This can without much of a stretch be cured by giving your pooch a lot of excellent vegan protein and healthy vegan meals.

Much the same as with yourself, it will be essential to keep an all-around organized and spread out meal plan for your canine so you can guarantee your closest companion is getting the best nutrition for ideal health.

6. Fishes and Animals do not Feel Pain

Who revealed this to you? Possibly toy fish and soft toys do not feel pain, yet any moving animals and fish surely feel torment.

Torment is not something exclusively human. The moment that an animal has nerves, it can feel torment, as nerves are the system that pain signals travel on. Do you believe it is an incident that in the event that you step on your canine's tail that they howl out?

7. It is Impossible to be Vegan if You Live or Travel Abroad. Eating Out as a Vegan Is Impossible!

Have you really gone outside of the country?

In numerous countries, it is EASIER to find vegan-accommodating dishes than it is back in the United States.

For instance, in the event that you travel to Thailand, India, Korea, or Hong Kong, you will be overpowered by the number of vegan choices accessible to you.

In the event that you travel to developing countries where food is rare, this is the place you may run into inconvenience. If you know in advance where you are venturing out, you can positively plan for it by connecting with expats previously living and working around there.

8. Soya (Soy) Is Destroying the Environment and the Rainforests

True and no.

True, the excess of soy crops is having a major influence on deforestation. Where do you think the soy is going?

Do you really believe that vegans are eating THAT much soy?

In all honesty, the soy crops that are causing widespread devastation of rainforests in South America and past are part of the meat business. Dairy animals, chickens, and fish are being sustained soy-based feed. Regardless, when you chomp into a cheeseburger, you are gnawing into a mouth loaded with soy. At the point when the dairy animals and chickens are eating only soy, everything returns round trip to us when we eat them.

In this way, indeed, soy crops are causing ecological harm, yet this is soy that is being created for slaughterhouse bovines and chickens, not for vegans.

Probably the ideal way you can help with preventing the ecological damage from soy crops is to quit eating meat. Ranchers will plant increasingly practical harvests if the interest is there. At this moment, the interest is centred on meat. You can change the world by changing what is on your plate.

9. Vegans Only Eat Processed Foods

While there are those people who are, in fact, vegan since they are eating only vegan generously processed foods, most vegans are not at all like that.

Most vegans are eating healthy, even meals that are pressed with crisp vegetables, organic products, grains, lentils, nuts, seeds, grows, superfoods, and substantially more.

Truly, there are a lot of vegan prepared foods; however, they are never the "standard" of veganism or a vegan diet. Truth be told, for most vegans, they do not believe them to be genuine vegan meals.

10. Veganism Is Impossible for Athletes, Your Workout Will Suffer

There are plenty of popular vegan athletes.

A vegan diet has been demonstrated on numerous occasions to be exceptionally successful for advancing the hard-hitting way of life of the world's first-class athletes. The myth that athletes cannot be champions AND vegans are extraordinarily silly.

11. You Need Meat For Muscle Building

Wrong once more. For reasons unknown, there is this thought that ONLY meat and animal products can give the protein and building squares required for first-class quality mass.

First of all, a vegan diet is PACKED with vegan protein. Some plant-based foods give more protein than animal sources!

Furthermore, vegan protein accompanies the additional advantage of an assortment of vitamins and nutrients, including cell reinforcements, which help fight free radicals in the body.

12. Tofu and Soy Contain Estrogen, which Lowers Testosterone and Gives You Cancer

We should get the realities straight here: Soy and soy-based tofu do not contain the real hormone, estrogen. On the off chance that they did, the side effects of overabundance estrogen would be clear on an overall scale, particularly for men.

Overall, soy contains isoflavones, which are exceptionally feeble phytoestrogens.

To call them phytoestrogens might be giving them a lot of credit. Isoflavones are estrogen-like, which implies they may impersonate not many of the attributes of real estrogen.

Beyond any doubt: Isoflavones are NOT estrogen.

Soy utilization, particularly fermented soy, has been demonstrated to be advantageous for human health. The catch, obviously, is moderate utilization.

13. Plantations Business Kills Many Animals

Some people pretend that the rural creation that goes into gathering the yields required for a vegan diet slaughters MORE animals every year than the animals that are murdered for utilization.

The truth is out; do people really believe that growing plants murders a larger number of animals than the business that is explicitly around to slaughter animals for food?

14. Vegan Diet Gives Less Energy

Again, have you at any point met a vegan?

Additionally, did you miss our instances of the vegan champion athletes?

We are not sure how this myth at any point began yet, in one way or another, the possibility that vegans have less energy because their diet is so severely advanced into the standard.

In the event that you converse with somebody who is really following a vegan diet with healthy vegan meals, you will see it is the polar opposite. Plant-based diets give you the nutrients you require for ideal working.

Furthermore, plant-based diets guarantee you do not have development of poisons from animal products. For instance, if you are not eating steaks or cheeseburgers, you do not need to worry over the anti-microbial and development hormone that is being injected into cows.

It is a direct result of their diets that vegans are probably the most energized people you will ever meet.

15. It Is Impossible to Be a Vegan Since Animal Products Are Everywhere

We can see how this myth feels genuine, as it truly seems like you will discover animal derivatives in pretty much everything. Indeed, even JELLO is produced using animals!

Indeed, even with the best intentions, manufacturers, eateries, and so on, they all commit errors. As a reaction, the industry puts forth a strong effort to distinguish genuinely vegan products.

In any case, this thought of vegan compulsiveness is not the best approach to take a gander at veganism.

Veganism is based on making a valiant effort. Being a vegan is based on settling on a cognizant decision not to hurt any animals. In all actuality, nobody is perfect. The purpose of veganism is that you try your closest to perfection to carry on with a real existence where you hold all life to be consecrated, and you show this through your actions.

You cannot control anybody yet yourself, and that is what is important.

16. We Should Worry About Other Problems in the World, not About Animals

I thoroughly concur... in light of the fact that that is actually what vegans do: They stress over huge issues affecting the world. Animals simply happen to be a part of it.

How are they part of it?

The greatest threat to humankind is the everyday natural demolition that is happening thanks to a great extent, partially to the breeding and farming industry.

From deforestation to contamination, these businesses are annihilating homes, lives, and the planet.

Vegans pick their way of life with an end goal to support animals, as well as the world overall. Vegans care about observing overall issues like starvation and contamination. THAT is the reason they decide to be vegan. Their way of life advances the renewal of the planet and the people on it.

17. People With Food Allergies Can not Be Vegans

This myth is exceptionally groundless. It is as a result of food hypersensitivities that numerous people decide to become vegan.

The best case of this is with those people who are lactose intolerant. The people who wind up with everyday indications of lactose narrow use, start looking for a diet that does not bring about those symptoms of swelling and consequent restroom trips.

The same is for people who have gluten intolerance. The street back to all normal, plant-based foods rapidly turns into the alternative for people with food hypersensitivities as they promptly report feeling better after doing the switch.

18. I Can not Be Vegan when My Family, Partner, or Roommate Is not

Actually, it is troublesome, yet it is certainly feasible.

The way to being vegan when your family, accomplice, or flatmate is not vegan is... communication!

Truly, it really is that easy. You need to communicate with the person or people you are living with. Tell them you are making a diet and lifestyle change, and you would appreciate it on the chance that they bolstered you.

They do not have to roll out the improvement, and you unquestionably do not have to change over them. They simply need to respect and back up your decisions.

In the event that somebody really cares about you, they will bolster your choice and make things as simple as possible for you.

Keep in mind; it is everything about being straightforward, comprehension, and approaching with thoughtfulness for help.

19. Being a Vegan Guarantees Weight Loss. Veganism Is Always Healthy

By pure chance, this myth is almost valid...

Actually, most of the devoted vegans you see are slim and fit as a fiddle; however, that does not mean EVERY vegan is unimaginably fit.

With the wide availability of processed vegan foods, it has never been simpler to have a horrible diet AND consider yourself a vegan.

Regardless of whether a vegan is eating only whole foods, exercise and legitimate segment control always are of major relevance. Calories will be calories all things considered.

CHAPTER 4

PROTEIN: MYTHS AND FACTS FOR ATHLETES

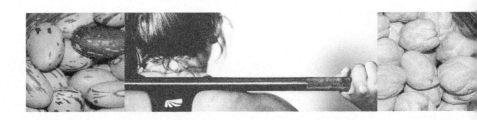

As a new vegan, you may receive inquiries concerning protein, which can be an issue since vegans, unlike other people, will be asked to give some information about their protein intake all the time; thus, many people get sick of responding to such inquiries. We understand the issue can be annoying, so let's find a few solutions!

1. The Need for Protein

Proteins are a wide scope of particles made up of building blocks called amino acids. At the point when we eat proteins, they are separated into singular amino acids and remade to frame the specific protein we need in the ideal spot.

The vast majority realize that muscles require loads of protein. However, all organs of the body require protein for general upkeep and for making new cells, as the body continually expels old cells and replaces them with new ones.

Proteins have a wide scope of capacities, for example, giving the "framework" of cells, putting cells together, shaping receptors on the outside of cells, which permits them to react to synthetic compounds, for example, hormones and controlling the action of qualities in DNA.

2. The Amount of Protein Needed for an Athlete

Rules given by institutions will, in general, instruct a day-by-day intake regarding around 55g for a grown-up. Another basic rule is around 0.8g of protein consumption for each kg of body weight.

Obviously, such rules are based on a "common grown-up"; thus may not really be ideal for your requirements yet are a decent spot to begin.

The rules are ordinarily based on a "sedentary" grown-up, which means somebody like, for instance, an office worker who just occasionally exercises.

Be that as it may, the prerequisites of people with exceptionally dynamic occupations and high-performance athletes are probably going to be higher, regular recommendations for consumption for such people extend between about 1.2-1.7g of protein per kg of body weight.

3. Is the Vegan Diet Protein Deficient?

The main thing is that nutrients provided by animal products are replaced by non-animal origin ones in vegan meals, after that, the substance of the meal is altogether up to the person.

Yet, there is no reason why removing meat from a diet should bring about protein-inadequacy. Basic staples of vegan and non-vegan diets still include grains, for example, rice and wheat, vegetables, for example, green peas and beans, nuts, and seeds, which are all high in protein.

On the off chance that meat-eaters imagine a vegan meal as their standard meat, veg, and potatoes yet without the meat, then you can comprehend why they may figure such a diet would be lacking in protein. Obviously, a vegan diet isn't just taking the meat off the plate, it's acquiring a whole scope of other food sources and supplements to make full, nutritious meals, and similarly, as with any diet, a vital aspect for making it healthy is to eat a scope of foods and to advantage from the various nutrients that different foods offer.

Among the vegan network are ultra-endurance athletes, tennis players, NFL players, NBA players, and a whole host of top-level athletes. Athletes push their bodies to limits of wellness, and numerous who settle on a vegan diet, regardless of whether for health or morals, proceed to flourish and improve truly. This goes to show there is nothing to state that a vegan diet should be insufficient in anything.

4. Is the Protein Gotten from Meat Better than the Protein Gotten Elsewhere?

Since most proteins are split down then developed again inside the body, the type of protein you eat doesn't make a difference. Many people think that eating meat, which is animal muscle, will help you with building muscle quicker because of the fact that you are eating muscle, but that is not how it works (for further evidence, look at the size of many of the vegan bodybuilders out there).

Anyway, there are some amino acids ("essential amino acids") which are not delivered by the body and are not present in any single vegan food. Hence supplanting meat in the diet should be done by expanding the intake of the scope of vegan foods to ensure all essential amino acids are secured.

For instance, two essential amino acids are lysine and methionine. Rice is high in methionine, while beans are high in lysine, so a meal or side-dish based on rice and beans (normal the world over and particularly well known among vegans as a modest, nutritious, delectable and simple to make a meal) easily satisfies your necessities.

5. Eating too Much / too Little Protein Causes Diseases

Protein inadequacy is a serious matter. Anyway, it happens mostly in those having an infection, the older, or citizens of developing countries. Among the industrialized world, protein inadequacy because of dietary lack (rather than increasingly regular protein insufficiencies brought about by hereditary qualities) is unbelievably low.

Issues may likewise happen from ingesting too much protein. The body cannot store overabundance of protein, so protein is utilized and discharged by the kidneys. This is fine except if you have an illness or you are taking medications which lessens your kidney work.

Numerous industries publications will list side effects of protein inadequacy, including tiredness, failure to rest, crankiness and food yearnings, all exceptionally broad indications which could be the aftereffect of an immense number of reasons. Yet such industries generally need to attempt to sell you a way of life or diet so will suggest that if you adhere to their guidelines your health will improve. We suggest that in the event that you have a genuine health issue you should contact your primary care physician as opposed to following the dubious guarantees of unknown people on the web.

6. What to Do if Protein Deficient?

In the event that you are feeling sick and suspect you might be inadequate in protein, it is ideal to consult your primary care physician, and they will presumably do a white blood cells test. Egg whites are cells in the blood utilized as a typical pointer of whole-body protein levels.

On the chance that you are feeling all right yet worried that your diet may not be satisfactory, at that point, you may need to investigate your diet. All the food you purchase should have visible nutritional data, so you should have the option to derive out, estimating the course of seven days, how much protein you are getting in your diet. On the off chance that it is lower than rule levels, or originates from an undetermined number of sources, then you may wish to increase the number and variety of protein-rich foods you eat.

7. The Vegan Protein Sources

Here is a rundown of some of my preferred protein sources and reasons why I like them.

Beans

Supplanting meat with beans is one of the most effortless and least expensive approaches regardless of a protein-rich vegan diet. There are such a large number of various assortments of beans available, in addition, meaning you can appreciate them from multiple points of view.

From white to dark beans, a legacy to pinto beans, they all contain a good parcel of protein. For example, you can get a significant pace of protein with only two cups of kidney beans. The best thing about beans is that they are truly adaptable and pair well with a lot of different foods. Who doesn't adore beans on toast, a major zesty pot of stew, or a bean burger?

You can likewise purchase beans in all forms - which kind of debunks that vegan food is hard to store in large quantities. Just as customary grocery supply, you can find extravagant, surprising or natural beans at supermarkets. Food supply is not different from health food supply. Great cash sparing tip is to get them dried in huge sacks and simply let them absorb water medium-term before cooking them. A jar of prepared beans covered with vegan cheddar and HP sauce is my definitive snappy, modest, comfort food.

Chickpeas

Chickpeas, also known as garbanzo beans, are legumes that can be cooked and eaten in heaps of ways. They are likewise a great addition to a plate of mixed greens. One-half cup of chickpeas contains around 7.3 grams of protein, and even sweeter, they are very low in calories while being high in fiber.

Green Peas

Like most foods that have a place with a group of vegetables, green peas are also acceptable sources of plant-based protein. Some of these peas contain about 7.9

grams of protein, which is about equivalent to some milk. In the event that you think that it is difficult to eat them as they are, you can mix them with other preparations, for example, adding them to a pesto sauce.

Nuts

A wide range of nuts, besides being a portion of the top veggie lover and vegan's sources of protein, are likewise good sources of healthy fats. This is the primary motivation behind why they are remembered continuously for a plant-based diet. One thing you have to remember, however, is that while they are delightful, nuts contain an incredible number of calories, especially pistachios, almonds, and cashews. It is important for you to go for either the dry simmered or the crude ones. Nut butter and almond spreads are likewise acceptable protein sources, anyway, be cautious in light of the fact that there are lots of brands that add a lot of sugar or hydrogenated oils.

Quinoa

Try not to worry too much over how you pronounce this one (it's 'keen waa'). Quinoa is a type of seed that many people see as a type of grain. This one of a kind food contains protein up to more than 8 grams/cup. Besides being a fantastic source of grain-based protein, it additionally has all the nine essential amino acids that your body needs to develop and fix itself. Its versatility is additionally astounding; you can add it to veggie bean stews and soups, eat it with products of fruit and minerals for breakfast, or add it into servings of mixed greens.

Tofu

Probably the most noteworthy vegan sources of protein are those that come from soybeans. Tofu and tempeh are two of the best examples. Tofu contains 40 grams for each cup, while Tempeh has 30 for every cup. Notwithstanding being impressively nutritious, these two have characteristics that permit it to take on the taste, yet additionally the texture of any type of food that one needs it to. There are tofu that are so delicate that you can without much of a stretch crush them with a fork (I like to utilize these to make cheesecake), and there are likewise firmer forms that can assume the characteristics of meat.

CHAPTER 5

NUTRITIONAL FACTS ABOUT VEGAN DIET

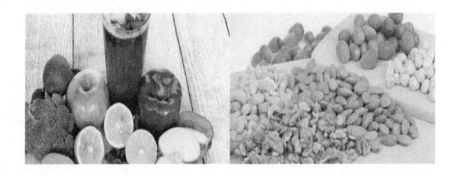

Counting calories and eating for weight loss, this one may say that is a thing, yet shouldn't something be said about basic nutrition? Your general nutrition is not only important for your health, yet it can likewise essentially affect how fertile you are. Furthermore, not getting the perfect or satisfactory amount of nutrients, can prompt any kind of inconvenience, from poor energy and performance to interminable ailment and other health conditions.

Getting appropriate nutrition is essentially the way of providing your body with the fundamental nutrients you need in order to stay healthy. Furthermore, nutrients are grouped into two classifications, based on the sum required by our bodies: macronutrients and micronutrients.

The two sets of nutrients give the whole of the essential components to advance our body's development and improvement and to control our body's functions. In any case, since everyone's body is different, it is imperative to recognize what the correct harmony between these nutrients is, for your body and for your specific goals.

Macronutrients

In the least complex definition, macronutrients are the components in food required for an individual to develop and work. They are required in huge amounts compared to other nutrients, which is the reason they are classified as macronutrients and are generally alluded to as "macros".

Macros give the whole of the calories you get from food and drinks.

For the most part, macronutrients are broken into three groups: sugars, protein, and fat. Alcohol is also viewed as a macro since it gives you calories. Yet, it is considered anything but an important source of nutrition, so it is regularly forgotten about when counting macros.

Every macro gives a different calorie sum for each gram - 4 grams for each calorie for protein and carbs, and 9 grams of calories for fat (alcohol gives 7 grams for every calorie). What's more, despite the fact that all macros give important energy, every macro has a different function in your body.

Since macros are essential, your calories should be put into key points. Figuring out how to adjust and track your macros is a well-known way to deal with weight loss and better wellness results.

Carbohydrates

We use carbohydrates for snappy energy - they are your body's preferred source of fuel since it does not take a ton of work to get energy from carbs. Our bodies effectively separate this macronutrient into glucose (sugar), which is a similar type of sugar found in your blood. Our cerebrums and muscles are the greatest users of glucose. However, all cells in our bodies use it to work. Anyway, the measure of carbs you need every day can vary, starting with one individual then onto the next based on an action level, weight, mass, general health, and so forth.

Notwithstanding, carbs are not essential for endurance. Your body has to work it out when carbs are not present for longer time frames, or conceivably perpetually, utilizing fat and protein. The keto diet works by these principles!

Likewise, not all carbs are created equal. Carbs originate from all plant-based foods and some dairy, yet they can likewise originate from straightforwardly from included sugar and many refined, unhealthy foods. Since carbs are so simple to get in the diet, they can, in general, get negative criticism. In any case, is advisable picking progressively healthy sources including whole grains, potatoes and tuberous, and beans, can improve your general nutrition and allow you to, in any case, be effective in getting more fit.

Sugars

All carbs are actually a type of sugar, however not every one of them acts the same about your health. Naturally present sugar, as the one found in organic products, milk, and vegetables, is frequently mistaken for added sugar. Sugar from whole foods will, in general, be mixed with other key nutrients and do not cause a relevant spike in glucose. However, added sugar will, in general, be found in, for the most part, refined foods, and when eaten alone (like in an industrial candy bar or soda) can unquestionably affect your energy and insulin levels more radically than other carbs.

As a general guideline, you should care to restrict added sugars and concentrate even more normally happening sources from plant-based foods.

Starches

Bland carbs are frequently alluded to as "mind-boggling carbs." This kind of carb brings the longest to separate, giving progressively supported energy and less effect on your glucose levels. This kind of food includes corn, beans, potatoes, and whole grains.

Fibres

What is more, finally, fiber! Numerous people do not really understand that fiber is a type of starch. Nevertheless, fiber is not as effortlessly processed, and cannot be consumed by the body, making it fundamentally unique in relation to other carb types. There are two primary kinds of fiber. Soluble fiber that helps draw with watering into your gut, supporting in sense of fullness, and favouring heart health (as it attracts water, it can likewise get cholesterol in addition to other things with it). Insoluble fiber that rather pushes everything through, supporting digestion and regularity.

The best sources of fiber include whole grains, beans, nuts, seeds, products of fruit and minerals.

Proteins

Protein is the "manufacturer" macro and not at all like carbs; is it essential for correct nutrition. Truth be told, protein assumes such a remarkable job; it is frequently your final retreat for day by day energy and rather used to construct, fix, and keep up your whole self.

We need protein in our diets since it furnishes us with essential amino acids that we cannot make ourselves. Our bodies resemble recycling masters that can take an old bed (plant and animal protein), separate it (into amino acids), and make a place from the parts (new protein). Proteins have an impact on the whole of our body's capacities from our sensory system to our digestive system, and our whole body, cells, DNA, and so on is totally composed of proteins.

Healthy protein sources include beans, nuts and seeds, lean meats, and eggs. In addition, keeping in mind that animal sources of protein have the most noteworthy protein content per calorie, you can likewise meet your protein needs without eating animal products on a vegan or veggie lover diet.

Fats

Fats, like protein, are an essential dietary must - they are a great long haul source of energy and furthermore do a fundamental job in keeping up healthy skin and hair, protecting body organs against decline, keeping up internal heat level, hormone guideline, and promoting healthy cell work.

Fat will, in general, get unfavourable criticism since it is the most calorie thick macro (giving more calories per volume). When eaten in abundance, it can without much of a stretch spoil the muscle to fat ratio. In any case, other macros can likewise spoil muscle to fat ratio, and this procedure expects you to eat a larger number of calories than you need - prompting weight gain. There is no compelling reason to fear fat as long as your calories are controlled, and you are utilizing a general macro balance that works for you.

Healthy vegan sources of fat include nuts and seeds, healthy oils, and avocados.

Saturated Fats

It is very discussed whether saturated fats are required, yet it broadly is commonly agreed we should not eat them in high quantities. While the researcher is uncertain about whether or not they are 100% "awful," high intakes of saturated fat have been related with expanded blood cholesterol in various investigations, and we have not found evident health benefits of this type of fat either.

Saturated fats are generally found in animal products like milk, cheddar, and meats, yet they are likewise found in littler sums in plant sources, for example, seeds and nuts, avocados, and plant oils.

Cholesterol

Cholesterol is a type of fat used to make hormones, Vitamin D, and digestion-related substances. However, it is not important to take in high measures of cholesterol because our bodies can produce it from the fat we eat. Research has likewise shown that dietary cholesterol may not be as firmly connected to blood cholesterol as we may once, however. Yet, it is presumably still advisable practice to avoid going over the edge.

Important dietary sources of cholesterol include cheddar, egg yolks, and greasy meats. It is not found in huge sums in plant sources.

Micronutrients

Called "micro" nutrients since they are required distinctly in extremely modest quantities, these substances do not give any calories however empower our bodies to deliver chemicals, hormones, and different substances imperative to improvement, malady prevention, and fertility.

Micronutrients are ordinarily alluded to as nutrients and minerals. In addition, it is a satisfactory intake of these micros that help lessen your danger of incessant sickness, advance a more extended life, and improve your general prosperity. Some researchers even demonstrate that higher intakes of micros are related to an improved state of mind, energy levels, and hunger control.

Pick an assortment of nutrient thick whole foods, similar to natural products, vegetables, whole grains, and lean proteins, to build your general intake of micros.

Getting the Right Nutrition for You

Largely, the primary goal of nutrition is to relate what you are eating to how it affects your body, particularly how your food is making you feel. In the event that you need to lose weight, have more energy, acquire muscle, and so forth, this is the basic thing you have to comprehend about your diet. Realizing what nutrition is best for you is a great beginning. In addition, monitoring how your diet explicitly affects your wellness goals and individual needs will spare you a great deal of undesirable worry over the long haul, permitting you to assume total responsibility for your health.

Step by step instructions to Count Macros

Counting macros is the way toward tracking what number of grams of each macronutrient you take in every day. What's more, since protein, fat, and carbohydrates each give a specific measure of calories per gram, you are additionally tracking what number of calories every day you take in.

Counting macros is a simple method to count calories and nutrients intake simultaneously.

When you know your calorie goals, you can without much of a stretch count your macros utilizing the following three stages:

Stage 1. Figure out How Many Calories per Macro

The calorie breakdown of your macros is as per the following:

Sugars and protein give approximately four calories for every gram - which means a food or drink with 10g of protein will give 40 calories from protein.

Fat is the most calorically thick nutrient and gives nine calories for every gram, so food or drink containing 10g of fat will give 90 calories from fat - more than double the measure of energy as protein and sugars.

Stage 2. Determine Total Macro Calories

You can determine the quantity you are eating by utilizing the nutritional properties label. It truly is that basic, anything that has a nutritional properties label, also has macronutrients shown. Truth be told, this is actually what the FDA uses to compute the measure of calories in your food.

Here is a case of the grain. A half-cup serving of this food gives 3 grams of fat, 13 grams of carbs, and 3 grams of protein.

In the event that you needed to additionally see what number of calories you are getting and the rate originating from every macro, you can multiply each sum by their assigned macronutrient carbohydrate content.

- 3g of fat x 9 calories for each gram = 27 calories

- 13g of carbs x 4 calories for each gram = 52 calories

- 3g of protein x 4 calories for each gram = 12 calories

These calorie sums consolidated should rise to the measure of all-out calories for the food - 90 calories for each serving!

Stage 3. Calculate Macro Ratio

To locate the macro proportion rate, you essentially divide every calorie sum by total calories (90) and afterwards multiply by 100.

Note: this rate is not quite the same as the per cent day-by-day esteem on the mark, which is taking a gander at your all-out day-by-day needs.

- 27 fat calories/90 calories x 100% = 30% of calories from fat

- 52 carb calories/90 calories x 100% = 57% of calories from carbs

- 12 protein fat calories/90 calories x 100% = 13% of calories from protein

The level of each one of the three - protein, fat and starches, should add up to 100%.

How many Macros Do You Need?

You can quickly decide your macro needs utilizing a spreadsheet that utilizes a progression of basic inquiries to survey your activity level and health goals.

On the other hand, you can generally assess your macros utilizing the straightforward equation underneath.

Step 1 - Choose your goal.

Are you trying to lose fat? build up muscle? On the other hand, would you like to keep up your weight as well as improve performance?

Step 2 - Calculate Calories

Estimate what number of calories you need every day to lose, gain, or keep up your weight. You can discover this utilizing a complete day-by-day energy consumption, using a software or a TDEE calculator.

Step 3 - Diagram

You can have a quick image of your macro needs utilizing this chart:

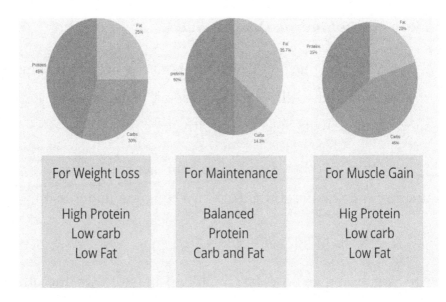

For Weight Loss	For Maintenance	For Muscle Gain
High Protein Low carb Low Fat	Balanced Protein Carb and Fat	Hig Protein Low carb Low Fat

Macro Diets

Obviously, it is not constantly a one-size-fits-all, and there are various adaptable dieting approaches you can use to control calories and equalize your nutrition by counting your carb, fat, as well as protein intake.

Therefore, whether you are a bodybuilder, or simply trying to eat healthier, here are some normal macro-based diet approaches you might have known about.

Weight Loss Macros

Starches are grasped in the athlete world. Macro planning and balance has been a mainstream device for upgrading performance and results, and this methodology can be applied to the average guy either. Seeing how carbs work and changing your intake of macronutrients to help your day-by-day needs about carbs, intense training as cycling or long-running might be an elective way to deal with simply disposing of carbs inside and out.

What is the amount of Protein needed to Lose Weight?

Protein is the most peculiar of a considerable number of macros since it is anything but a preferred source of energy and is to the least extent liable to be put away as muscle to fat ratio. Protein likewise keeps up fit muscle takes more energy to process (more thermogenic than different macros) and it should help control craving and decrease hunger.

Muscle Gain Macros

Putting on a healthy weight requires a vital macro and preparing centre. Find a workable pace on the perfect macros for building muscle, and ensure you stick to those gym workout days you set.

Keto Diet Macros

Are you experiencing difficulty adhering to a lower fat intake? Consider switching things up with a high fat, low carb diet for weight loss like keto.

Vegan Macros

Since plants are regularly a source of carbs and fats, exploring a high protein, plant-based diet can feel challenging.

Macro Meal Planning

When you have your macronutrient proportions dialled in, you can plan your day-by-day meal plan around them.

Here are the means by which to construct a strong menu to get your goals:

Start by realizing which healthy foods include each macronutrient.

Then get acquainted with gauging and assign your food with these partition guidelines.

Learn to meal prep like if you are your own supervisor, to measure your macros and eat the foods you love most.

Track your day-by-day consumption utilizing a food tracking application.

Vegan Protein

It is normally considered that vegans do not get enough protein in their diet or that they really need more protein than meat-eaters.

Whether you are eating meat or not, your protein needs are unequivocally determined by your movement level, health and wellness goals, and absolute calorie consumption. Generally, you should most likely be endeavouring to get at any rate 25 to 30g of protein per meal or 1g of protein per pound of slender weight.

The issue with plant-based sources is that they are commonly a source of carbs or fat too – nuts contain protein, yet in addition, contain a lot of fat, and keeping in mind that beans are a decent source of protein, they are likewise reasonably high on the carb. Lamentably, this will, in general, be the situation with every plant-based protein you can consider.

High Protein Foods for Vegans

So which vegan proteins are going to give you the most value for your money?

For researchers, here is the macro breakdown of regular protein-containing foods and a glance at what 100 calories of each will get you:

Food	Protein (G)/100 Cal	Carb (G)/100 Cal	Fat (G)/100 Cal
Egg Whites	22g	1.5g	0.5g
Grass-bolstered steak	20g	0g	2g
Chicken Breast	19g	0g	2.5g
Low Fat Yogurt	13g	5g	3g

Salmon	11g	0g	6g
Tofu	12g	4g	4g
Tempeh	11g	4g	6g
Edamame	10g	7g	3.5g
Soy Veggie Burger	9g	8g	3.5g
Lentils	8g	17g	0g
Green Peas	7g	17g	0.5g
Dark Beans	7g	18g	0g
Peanuts	4.5g	2g	8.5g
Quinoa	3.5g	18g	1.5g

Reference: https://ndb.nal.usda.gov/ndb/

Tofu and soy-based choices will, in general, be your best food alternative, as they contain moderately low carbs and fat and are a decent source of value protein.

In case you are not enthusiastic about soy, food makers continually see approaches to grow more protein choices for plant-based diets. Knowing precisely what to look for can help you with amplifying your decisions as needed. Some promoted choices may sound great, yet at the same time need basic nutrition, or they are intensely refined. A few veggies burgers are not even a decent source of protein (5g or more) and can be full of fat.

Here are important things you will need to consider while looking at some vegan "meat" choices from the store:

- Vegan meats should generally have 40% of their calories originating from protein or 10g of protein for every 100 calories.

- Check the fat and carbs to ensure the alternatives fit inside your macro range. Lean proteins will have under 8g of fat per serving. Furthermore, adequate carb choices should have under 25g of carbs per serving.

- Read the label and look for alternatives that are less prepared and contain quality proteins.

Getting Complete Protein

When you eat, your body separates protein into amino acids that are utilized for different tasks- like building, fixing, and healing muscle The rest of them are utilized for energy. Your body can make some amino acids by itself, however, other kinds you can only get from food. Nine amino acids are viewed as essential in the diet because your body needs them, yet cannot deliver them.

Numerous sources of plant-based protein are not considered "total" since they do not contain sufficient quantities of all essential amino acids you need to stay healthy. This is the reason numerous sources of nutrition guidance disclose to us that you should take in all essential amino acids in a single meal, through corresponding protein alternatives that equivalent satisfactory amino acid intake, to get what's known as a "total protein."

In any case, do not stress at this time, things being what they are, following a diet containing the whole of your essential amino acids for the duration of the day might be adequate. Furthermore, your body can fill in any holes with free amino acids available through typical protein breakdown and recycling. At the end of the day, on the off chance that you do not get the whole of your amino acids in sufficient amounts each and every day, your body has methods for trading off to get you what you need - as long as you are following a fair diet.

About building up the mass, nevertheless, the type of protein you are eating might be important. Studies recommend that animal protein is more anabolic than plant protein because of their amino acid substance - which means they bolster building muscle all the more effectively. While the exploration of taking a gander at animal versus plant protein is still genuinely constrained, eating a total or corresponding protein during your dynamic recuperation window, 20 minutes after a workout, could be progressively gainful when it comes to building and fixing muscle.

Picking proteins should improve largely absorption and decrease the requirement with the expectation of complementary amino acid use. At the end of the day, your body will not need to fill in as difficult to get the correct muscle-building amino acids after a workout when you are consuming them on the spot, which permits you to recoup even more proficiently.

Based on acid amino balance, here are the best vegan protein combos; you can eat to get a total protein:

- Soy Protein Isolate

- Rice + Peas

- Whole Grains + Legumes

- Grains + Vegetables

- Grains + Nuts + Seeds

- Legumes + Nuts + Seeds

Vegan Protein Absorption

It is, to some degree, genuine that some plant-based proteins are not as bioavailable for absorption by the body compared with meat and dairy. This contention originates from something many refer to as the Protein Digestibility Corrected Amino Acid Score (PDCAAS). PDCAAS was received by the Food and Agriculture Organization of the United Nations (FAO) as an estimation of protein quality in surveying world hunger. What's more, subsequently, it has been utilized as a pointer of protein quality from that point onward.

Taking a gander at the PDCAAS, one would expect you could wind up avoiding 30% of the protein from plants because of poor absorbability. Nevertheless, fortunately, the FDA requires nutrition naming to address this, and what you see on the label is what you really get.

In case you are interested at any rate, here is what the study shows as far as PDCAAS for basic proteins:

Food Protein Digestibility Percentage

Food	%
Dairy	100%
Eggs	100%
Mycoprotein	99%
Soy	98%
Beef	98%
Quinoa	91%
Edamame and Chickpeas	88%
Lentils	84%
Dark Beans	72%
Vegetables	73%

Green Peas	59%
Peanuts	52%

Best Protein Powder for Vegans

As a last resort, supplements can be a simple method to take in a lot of protein without additional carbs and calories. Powders are made by concentrating only the protein segment of certain plant-based foods to give you generally 20g of protein for around 100 calories – making them a great nutrient supplement.

While customary whey and casein do not fit into a vegan diet, there are many finished, top-notch choices available. Soy protein concentrate is frequently commended as the best alternative, however different mixes of rice and pea, just as spirulina, can be just as much acceptable.

Carb Cycling on a Vegan Diet

Since starches originate from whatever comes out of the ground, plant-based diets will, in general, be very substantial in carbs. This can be great about sustenance, yet not that good when you are trying to burn fat by cutting carbs or simply decline your carb intake during rest periods.

If you are picking a protein source that is additionally light in carbs, you should modify your starch partitions as needed, and settle on "non-boring" veggies or low carb organic products. While beans and quinoa give a great protein combo, to find a workable pace, you will likewise be taking in more than 600 calories and 100 grams of carbs. Contrasted with 30g of protein from vegan-steak, which is under 200 calories and 0g of carbs.

To help counteract a portion of this, you can generally settle on your starch, using it likewise as a source of protein. Furthermore, non-bland veggies and low carb organic products should fill the rest of your plate to include nutrition without an excessive number of carbs or extra calories.

The following is a proposed macro plan based on your performance and weight loss goals. How about we investigate how you can figure out how to take your food decisions to hit your vegan macros targets.

Step 1: Choose a protein-rich carb choice like quinoa, beans, peas, or lentils.

Step 2: Choose a nutrient thick protein choice like tofu or a vegan "meat".

Step 3: Combine the carb and protein utilizing integral proteins, or nutrient thick vegan proteins, and scale back.

Here's a proposed breakdown:

- Maintain: half veggie/natural product, half vegan protein blend
- Gain Muscle: 40% veggie/natural product, 60% vegan protein blend
- Lean Out: 60% veggie, 40% vegan protein blend (choose generally low carb/thick nutrient proteins on nowadays)

Healthy Fats for Vegans

You may have noticed that fat is not referenced in the plan above, why this?

Fats are normally utilized as condiments or, sometimes, happen to naturally be in certain foods, so there is not a need to include an assigned part at every meal – you likely experience little difficulty getting enough fat into your day. In any case, this could likewise be a chance to get a little protein support with things like nuts and nut spreads, seeds, and nutritional yeast.

On the chance that you are trying to control calories, cutting fat is a simple method to cut calories without reducing the servings too much. Albeit, a tad of fat is important for satiety and nutrient absorption.

CHAPTER 6

VEGAN ATHLETES FOOD FOR WORKOUT

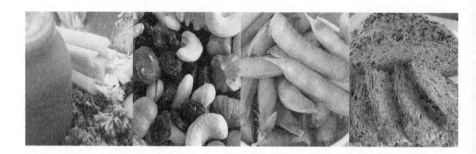

Vegan Grocery List

This is what a standard shopping list resembles. A couple of things you clearly do not purchase inevitably, yet they are acceptable to keep around for cooking.

- Fruit: Apples, Oranges, Bananas, Pineapples, Mixed Frozen Berries (for smoothies), Lemons, Limes, Tomatoes, Avocados

- Vegetables: Romaine Lettuce, Spinach, Broccoli, Kale, Celery, Cucumbers, Bell Peppers, Jalapeno Peppers, Onions, Carrots, Garlic, Basil, Parsley, Cilantro

- Starchy Vegetables: Potatoes, Sweet Potatoes

- Legumes: Lentils, Chickpeas, Black Beans (preferably dry, however canned are ok)

- Non-Wheat Grains: Brown Rice, Quinoa (not, in fact, a grain), Granola, Spelt Pasta

- Wheat Products (limited): Whole-Wheat Bread, Pasta, Pitas, Bagels, and Wraps

- Breakfast Cereals: Post Grape Nuts (pressed with sugars), Kashi

- Nuts and Seeds: Almonds, Cashews, Walnuts, Flaxseeds

- Spreads and Pastes: Hummus, Nut Butters (almond is great however costly), Tahini (sesame seed glue), Baba Ganoush

- Oils: Olive Oil, Grapeseed Oil, Toasted Sesame Oil, Flaxseed Oil, Coconut Oil (strong at room temperature, regularly in the health food path

- Vinegar: Apple Cider Vinegar, Balsamic Vinegar

- Protein powder: Hemp (found in health store)

- Soy Products (limited): Tofu, Tempeh, Soy Sauce or Bragg's Amino Acids

- Tea and Coffee (limited)

- Other Snacks (limited): Tortilla Chips, Salsa, Popcorn

- Miscellaneous: Almond Milk, Coconut Milk, Agave Nectar (as workout fuel, not a regular use sugar), Honey (not strictly vegan but many vegans use it)

Furthermore, in case you are willing to eat non-meat animal products, as a rule, or while transitioning to a fully vegan diet:

- Eggs

- Milk, Yogurt, Cheese

Pre Workout Vegan Meals

By all accounts, when it comes to how, if and what to eat up before a workout, everyone has their own opinion. Would it be advisable for me to make a protein shake? Have a few organic products? Do I, at any point, need anything by any means? Eventually, everybody is different, and we as a whole have distinctive nutritional needs—so give a couple of these "unintentionally vegan" workout foods a shot and find your ideal blend.

For your pre-workout tidbit or meal, ensure that you are getting something with complex sugars to give you the energy for that additional set—however, keep it light, so stomach cramps do not intrude on your workout!

Nut Fruits and Butter

An apple or a banana will give you a decent spurt of energy before your workout. Bananas are stacked with potassium, which will help prevent muscle cramps and recharge the potassium that you lose when you sweat. Toss in some nut butter for an eruption of protein and enduring energy for long or extraordinary workouts.

Oats with Fruit, Nuts, or Chia Seeds

Oats are great since they are resistant starches that give a dependable source of energy. Do not hesitate to include some natural products for a snappy explosion of energy, a bunch of nuts for protein, or some chia seeds for a huge amount of additional health benefits.

Dried Fruit with a Handful of Almonds and Walnuts

The unsweetened dried organic fruit can be an astounding source of healthy sugars, and when matched with a bunch of nuts, they can be an ideal pre-workout nibble for any individual who is in a hurry or has restricted time.

Whole Grain Toast

Whole grain bread will give you the energy that you have to use through your workout. On the chance that you have an hour or two preceding your workout, include some almond spread or avocado to your toast for extra nutrients and supported energy. Simply recollect that these additions will take more time for your body to process.

Sweet Potato

Sweet potatoes have since a long time ago been viewed as a superfood for sprinters, and it might be the ideal opportunity for different athletes to add them into their meals before working out. They are a magnificent complex starch that is stacked with nutrients and minerals—which will help you with accomplishing your goals on the training ground.

Espresso

This one is kind of a weirdo, however, espresso, has been connected to expanded performance at the gym. In addition, its diuretic impact is negligible and is counteracted by the fluid found in the espresso itself. In case you are going after a beverage 30 minutes to an hour prior to your workout, consider making it some dark espresso—you can likewise include a light measure of soy or almond milk to it.

Pretzels

Pretzels can be a speedy and convenient approach to fuel up on carbs before hitting the gym. Plunge the pretzels in almond butter for some extra protein and support energy all through your workout.

Post-Workout Vegan Meal

In the event that you, despite everything, think vegans have some hard time being fit and healthy, it is an ideal opportunity to show some signs of life. Regardless of whether they are crushing world records in endurance or weight lifting, winning bodybuilding competitions, or bringing home UFC titles, the decision is in: Muscles don't need to worry about meat.

So a great deal of carbs, a better than average measure of protein (Ideally says 6 to 20 grams), bunches of cancer prevention agents, and minimal fat? If that is not vegans' main thing best, we do not have the foggiest idea what is.

Whenever you need to nourish your muscles right, you cannot fall flat with one of these recipes.

1. Teriyaki Mushrooms and Broccoli Soba Noodles

Produced using buckwheat, soba noodles have that 4:1 proportion, but on the other hand, they are a finished protein. Add to the Japanese noodles some teriyaki mushrooms for a rich, fulfilling, meaty recipe, just as broccoli and bean stews, which have anti-inflammatory properties. Cruciferous vegetable intake attenuates circling levels of pro-inflammatory markers in women.

2. Lentil and Spinach Soup

Well known for what it's worth, the 4:1 proportion of carbs to protein is not gospel. A few people prefer something closer to 2:1 or 3:1, and there are other people who think you'll recoup fine and dandy with just carbs and no protein by any stretch. Universal Society of Sports Nutrition position stand: nutrient planning.

3. Cherry Oats Chocolate

With their dietitian-endorsed 4:1 proportion, oats are a great decision, in spite of their protracted prep time. The enchantment of slow cooking comes in. This recipe is perfect post-workout because of the combo of cocoa powder, an incredible calming operator, and fruits, which help lessen post-workout muscle irritation.

4. Chickpea, Mango, and Curried Cauliflower Salad

Chickpeas have a 3:1 proportion, which combined with their practically complete absence of fat, makes them a great choice for refuelling post-workout. This present plate of mixed greens' dressing is a perfect nibble, and the spinach and lime juice give vitamin C to help your body with absorbing the muscle-accommodating iron in the chickpeas.

5. Quinoa-Stuffed Poblano Peppers

With its estimable use of beans, peppers, onions, and cancer prevention agent rich herbs, bona fide Mexican food can be pretty vegan inviting (simply hold the cheddar, obviously, and ensure the beans and tortillas aren't prepared with animal fat). This recipe puts a new twist on a conventional Southwestern dish with the expansion of in vogue quinoa, which, when mixed with protein-rich dark beans, has a great balance of carbs and complete protein.

6. Smooth Asparagus and Pea Soup

Pea protein is quickly turning into a famous supplement for vegans and non-vegans because of its elevated levels of branched-chain amino acids and the way that it is lactose and gluten-free, making it simple to process and hypersensitivity friendly. Pea protein oral supplementation advances muscle thickness gains during training according to a double-blind, randomized, Placebo-controlled clinical study comparing it with Whey protein.

7. Matcha Mango Chia Seed Pudding

Modest as they seem to be, chia seeds are a complete protein, and in spite of the fact that they may contain more fat than the ideal post-workout nibble (there's about twice as much fat as there is protein), they're as yet a good choice. The greater part of the fats are omega-3 unsaturated fats, and while people have some harder time retaining plant-based omega-3s than those found in animal sources, chia seeds are as yet a fantastic anti-inflammatory food. Alpha-Linolenic acid supplementation and transformation to n-3 long-chain polyunsaturated unsaturated fats in people.

8. Wild Rice and Broccoli Salad with Edamame

Edamame — those soybeans many people eat before sushi, mostly for killing time — are about a great balance of protein and carbs. This plate of mixed greens gives its best with a dynamic mix of broccoli, peas, and raisins. Double the bit for a delightful yet light meal.

9. Chickpea Sunflower Sandwich

A classic, the sandwich is a post-workout weapon of choice since it is so easy to make and pack in a gym bag.

10. Butternut Squash and Tempeh Tacos

Tempeh has twice the number as much protein as sugars, so wrench up your carbs with the addition of butternut squash. The warming flavours in the tempeh pair splendidly with the squash's sweetness. Furthermore, do not forget the handcrafted salsa Verde: It is stuffed with fiery cell reinforcements from tomatillos, onions, jalapeño, and cilantro.

11. Red Lentil Dal

A fundamental staple from a country with more than a billion vegans, this thick, protein-rich soup is produced using major dal or red lentils. These cook importantly quicker than the green kind; however, the nutrition profile is generally the equivalent. Dal is cherished as a solace food to some degree since it is generally made with a liberal measure of ghee or fat. To keep things animal-free, this recipe utilizes coconut milk, which implies your meal should process somewhat more rapidly in the event that you utilize the light form.

12. Apple Ginger Green Smoothie

How can you consider the post-workout meal finished without a protein shake? Smoothies are an extremely simple approach to pack a huge amount of foods with various health benefits into one simple to-chug bundle, and this recipe does not disillusion. It has calming benefits from ginger, and the calcium from kale and parsley may help with fat loss and lift muscle-building testosterone. Alkaloids and athlete safe capacity: caffeine, theophylline, gingerly, ephedrine, and their congeners. It is difficult to nail down a precise macronutrient proportion for a shake since it relies largely upon the type of protein powder you use, so it merits trying different things with various recipes to locate your most loved go-to combo.

13. Simmered Red Pepper Hummus

This hummus recipe is based on tahini, lemon squeeze, and simmered red pepper for its flavour. Not exclusively is delectable produce directly into the hummus itself, but at the same time, it is an ideal dip for any vegetable (in the event that you need to build your cell reinforcements) or pita bread (on the chance that you would prefer to finish your protein and include some extra carbs).

14. Dark Bean Sweet Potato Chili

No meat does not mean any bean stew for vegans. This rich, thick, velvety, zesty, and sweet mixture hits quite a few notes, and albeit dark beans have less than 3 grams of carbs for each gram of protein, that is just one of the methods that permit you to enjoy that warm, comforting sweet potato.

CHAPTER 7

A 4 WEEKS VEGAN MEAL PLAN

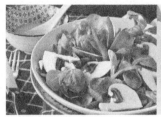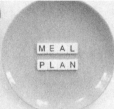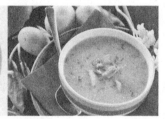

Week One

DAY 1

Breakfast: Vanilla chia pudding with 1 cup of fresh berries

Lunch: Crunchy red cabbage and green apple and sesame slaw with 1 cup of steamed, cubed sweet potato.

Snack: 1/4 cup hemp hummus with fresh vegetables (carrots, celery, romaine leaves, pepper, etc.)

Supper: Black bean and quinoa serving of mixed greens in with cumin dressing

Dessert: Dark chocolate

DAY 2

Breakfast: Smoothie with 1 cup of almond milk, 1 banana, 1-2 tbsps almond spread, one serving of protein powder, and a heaping cup of green leaves vegetables (spinach, chard, kale, etc.).

Lunch: one dark rice tortilla (Food for Life brand has a good one) or two without gluten corn tortillas with 1/4 cup hemp hummus, new or seared red ringer pepper, cut cucumbers, and many greens. Serve with steamed vegetables if preferred, or a little side plate of mixed greens.

Snack: Vegan protein bar

Supper: Zucchini Pasta with Cherry Tomatoes, Sweet Potato, Basil, and Hemp "Parmesan"

Dessert: Banana Bread

DAY 3

Breakfast: Quinoa breakfast porridge with 1 cup fresh berries

Lunch: Large plate of mixed greens in with three cups of greens, whichever veggies you like, 3 tbsps pumpkin or hemp seeds, and a dressing of choice (from the dressing options in the list).

Snack: 4 tbsps hemp hummus with fresh vegetables (carrots, celery, romaine leaves, ringer pepper, etc.)

Supper: Small prepared sweet potato with a tbsp of coconut oil, a huge bit of common dim beans, and steamed greens as needed (or a fresh side serving of mixed greens)

Dessert: 2 unrefined brownie snack

DAY 4

Breakfast: Peanut Butter and Chocolate Chip Nirvana bar, new natural item plate of mixed greens as preferred

Lunch: Kale plate of mixed greens in with 1/2 cup chickpeas

Snack: 1 oz. almonds and two or three tbsps raisins

Supper: White bean and summer vegetable pasta (serve with quinoa or dull shaded rice pasta)

Dessert: 2 unrefined vegan vanilla macaroons

DAY 5

Breakfast: Smoothie with 1 cup almond milk, 1 cup set blueberries, 1 serving chocolate Nutrition protein, 3 tbsps of hemp seeds, and 1 cup green leaves vegetables of choice

Lunch: The leftover white bean and the summer vegetable pasta or a gigantic green serving of mixed greens in with a huge part of a cup of beans or lentils, two tbsps cut almonds, vegetables based on your own preference, and turmeric tahini dressing

Snack: Apple with 2 tbsps almond margarine

Supper: Butternut squash curry served multiple/2 cup cooked quinoa, steamed vegetables as needed

Dessert: Dark chocolate

DAY 6

Breakfast: Banana and almond butter oats (equation to follow)

Lunch: Smoky avocado and jicama serving of mixed greens

Snack: 1 cup almond milk blended in with Nutrition protein powder and several ice strong shapes

Supper: Black bean and corn burgers, served with a bit of serving of mixed greens or steamed vegetables

Dessert: two rough vegan vanilla macaroons.

DAY 7

Breakfast: Smoothie of 1/2 dried banana, 1 cup peach compote, 2 ice cubes, 3/4 cup almond milk, 1 cup green leaves vegetables, and 1 serving Nutrition vanilla protein powder

Lunch: Leftover dim bean and corn burger, a small serving of mixed greens

Snack: 1/4 cup vegan trail mix of choice (or 2 tbsp. rough almonds or cashews and 2 tbsp. dried natural item)

Supper: One cup cooked quinoa, darker rice, or millet, served with 1/2 cut avocado, 1 cup steamed greens, and dressing of choice .

Dessert: 1/2 cup Choco mole

Week Two

DAY 8

Breakfast: sans gluten banana hotcakes, served with 1 cup fresh berries

Lunch: Mango, kale, and avocado serving of mixed greens

Snack: Apple, banana, melon, berries, or some other fresh fruit of choice

Supper: Eggplant with cashew cheddar, steamed greens or broccoli as needed

Dessert: Dark chocolate

DAY 9

Breakfast: Apple cinnamon oatmeal

Lunch: Roasted butternut squash and apple soup, served with a fresh green plate of mixed greens or steamed veggies as needed

Snack: Nutrition bar

Supper: Raw zucchini alfredo with basil and cherry tomatoes, served with another serving of mixed greens or steamed vegetables as needed

Dessert: 2 rough vegan brownie snack

DAY 10

Breakfast: Smoothie of 1 cup fresh blueberries or mixed berries, 1 cup coconut water, 1/2 small avocado, 1 serving Chocolate protein powder, and a scramble of cinnamon.

Lunch: Curried yellow lentils with avocado bread trims

Snack: Fresh vegetable crudités with 1/4 cup hemp hummus

Supper: Black bean and quinoa plate of mixed greens in with smart cumin dressing

Dessert: 1/2 cup Choco mole

DAY 11

Breakfast: 1 cut banana with 1 cup regular puffed rice or millet grain

Lunch: Kale Salad with Apples, Raisins, and Creamy Curry Dressing

Snack: 1/4 cup rough mix of choice

Supper: Sweet Potato Lime Burgers, new serving of mixed greens or steamed vegetables as needed

Dessert: two rough vanilla macaroons.

DAY 12

Breakfast: Vanilla chia pudding with 1 cup new berries

Lunch: Red quinoa, almond, and arugula plate of mixed greens in with melon

Evening Snack: a few rough nutty spreads and jam snack balls

Supper: Sweet potato and dim bean stew with steamed broccoli or greens

Dessert: 1/2 cup Choco mole

DAY 13

Breakfast: Smoothie of 1 banana, 1/2 cup mango compote, 1 stacking cup spinach leaves, 1 cup coconut water, and 1/2 avocado

Lunch: Bowl of staying dim bean and sweet potato stew with a small serving of mixed greens or steamed greens

Snack: Nutrition bar of choice

Supper: Cauliflower rice with lemon, mint, and pistachios, served over new greens

Dessert:Spicy almond milk hot cocoa.

DAY 14

Breakfast: Banana and almond spread oats

Lunch: Carrot avocado bisque with fiery Thai plate of mixed greens

Snack: Raw vegetable crudités with sweet potato hummus

Supper: Brown rice and lentil plate of mixed greens, served with another serving of mixed greens or steamed vegetables as needed and dressing of choice

Dessert: 2 unrefined vanilla macaroons

Week Three

DAY 15

Breakfast: Strawberry ginger chia pudding

Lunch: Leftover brown rice and lentil plate of mixed greens, served with a big mixed vegetable serving of mixed greens and dressing of choice.

Snack: 2 nutty spread and jam snack balls

Supper: Raw nut noodles with steamed vegetables or new serving of mixed greens as needed

Dessert: Dark chocolate

DAY 16

Breakfast: Smoothie with 1 cup of the almond milk, 1 banana, 1-2 tbsps almond spread, one serving of protein powder, and a stacking cup of green leaves vegetables (spinach, chard, kale, etc.)

Lunch: Mango, kale and avocado serving of mixed greens

Snack: Vegetable crudités as needed and 1/4 cup hemp hummus

Supper: Un-burned dull hued rice and vegetables

Dessert: 2 crudes, vegan brownie eats

DAY 17

Breakfast: Banana breakfast wraps

Lunch: The brown rice tortilla "pizza" and a side plate of mixed greens

Snack: Nutrition bar

Supper: Arugula plate of mixed greens in with cooked oak seed squash, goji berries, and cauliflower

Dessert: Delicate Banana serve

DAY 18

Breakfast: Apple cinnamon oatmeal

Lunch: Fennel, avocado, and tomato plate of mixed greens in with 1/2 cup chickpeas or white beans

Snack: 1 cup almond milk blended in with Protein Powder

Supper: Roasted vegetable pesto pasta plate of mixed greens

Dessert: Dark chocolate

DAY 19

Breakfast: sans gluten, vegan pumpkin scones with a tbsp of almond margarine and an apple

Lunch: The Kale Salad with Apples, Raisins, and Creamy Curry Dressing; 1 cup stewed cauliflower and parsnip soup

Snack: 1/3 cup unrefined way mix of choice (or a mix of rough almonds and raisins or goji berries)

Supper: Raw marinated Portobello mushroom "steak" and cauliflower "pureed potatoes," served with steamed greens or broccoli

Dessert : Blueberry ginger solidified yogurt

DAY 20

Breakfast: Smoothie of 1 cup hardened blueberries or mixed berries, 1 cup coconut water, 1/2 minimal avocado, 1 serving Chocolate protein powder, and a scramble of cinnamon

Lunch: Easy curried yellow lentils with avocado, served with a plate of mixed greens and dressing of choice or steamed vegetables as needed

Snack: Celery sticks served with 2 tbsps of nut or almond spread and raisins ("ants on a log" style)

Supper: Dish of mixed greens of rough greens and vegetables of picking, 1 cup cooked sweet potato, 1/2 avocado, cubed, ½ cup cooked lentils, and a dressing of choice from the recipe.

Dessert: 2 vegan brownie eats

Week Four

DAY 21

Breakfast: 1 cut banana and new berries with 1 cup normal puffed rice or millet oat (I like Arrowhead Mills brand) and 1 cup almond milk

Lunch: Smoky avocado and jicama plate of mixed greens, 1 little apple at whatever point needed

Snack: 2 nutty spread and jam snack balls

Supper: Butternut squash curry served multiple/2 cup cooked quinoa, steamed vegetables as needed

Dessert: Dark chocolate.

DAY 22

Breakfast: Smoothie of 1 set banana, 1/2 cup set mango, 1 stacking cup spinach leaves, 1 cup coconut water, and 1/2 avocado

Lunch: Leftover quinoa enchilada, a side plate of mixed greens in with the dressing of choice

Snack: Nutrition bar of choice

Supper: Sweet potato and dim bean stew with steamed broccoli or greens

Dessert: two unrefined vegan vanilla macaroons.

DAY 23

Breakfast: Vanilla chia pudding with 1 cup fresh berries

Lunch: Red quinoa, almond, and arugula plate of mixed greens in with melon

Snack: a few rough nutty spreads and jam snack balls

Supper: Sweet potato and dim bean stew with steamed broccoli or greens

Dessert: 1/2 cup Choco mole

DAY 24

Breakfast: Smoothie of 1 banana, 1/2 cup set mango, 1 heaping cup spinach leaves, 1 cup coconut water, and 1/2 avocado

Lunch: Bowl of staying dull bean and sweet potato stew with a small serving of mixed greens or steamed greens

Snack: Nutrition bar of choice

Supper: Cauliflower rice with lemon, mint, and pistachios, served over new greens

Dessert: Spicy almond milk hot cocoa

DAY 25

Breakfast: Smoothie with 1 cup of almond milk, one big banana, 1-2 tbsps almond spread, one serving of protein powder, and a stacking cup of green leaves vegetables (spinach, chard, kale, etc.)

Lunch: One dull shaded rice tortilla (Food for Life brand) or two without gluten corn tortillas with 1/4 cup hemp hummus, fresh or stewed red ringer pepper, cut cucumbers, and many greens. Present with steamed vegetables as needed, or a little side plate of mixed greens.

Snack: Nutrition bar

Supper: Farro salad, almond, avocado and arugula

Dessert: Banana bread.

DAY 26

Breakfast: Apple cinnamon oatmeal

Lunch: Roasted butternut squash and apple soup, served with another green plate of mixed greens or steamed veggies as needed

Snack: Nutrition bar

Supper: Raw zucchini alfredo with basil and cherry tomatoes, served with another plate of mixed greens or steamed vegetables as needed

Dessert: 2 rough vegan brownie eats

DAY 27

Breakfast: Smoothie of 1 cup hardened blueberries or mixed berries, 1 cup coconut water, 1/2 minimal avocado, 1 serving Chocolate protein powder, and a scramble of cinnamon.

Lunch: Easy curried yellow lentils with avocado bread trims

Snack: Fresh vegetable crudités with 1/4 cup hemp hummus

Supper: Black bean and quinoa plate of mixed greens in with energetic cumin dressing

Dessert: 1/2 cup Choco mole

DAY 28

Breakfast: Vanilla chia pudding with 1-cup new berries.

Lunch: Crunchy red cabbage and green apple sesame slaw with 1 cup steamed, cubed sweet potato (or 1 minimal sweet potato, prepared)

Snack: 1/4 cup hemp hummus with fresh vegetables (carrots, celery, romaine leaves, toll pepper, etc.)

Dessert: Dark chocolate

Nutrition Guide and Sources of Nutrients

We can get all the important nutrients we need without eating animal products.

An even vegan diet can give numerous health benefits, is appropriate for all ages and can altogether bring down the danger of basic health issues, for example, coronary illness, stroke, diabetes, weight, hypertension, elevated cholesterol, and disease.

Protein

Protein is an important nutrient for development and has numerous capacities all through the body, including being an important segment of muscles. Protein is made out of substances called amino acids. There are 20 distinctive amino acids we require for protein amalgamation, yet just 9 of these are viewed as essential as our bodies can't make these; thus, these should be given in our diet.

Protein sources – Virtually all foods contain protein, and vegans can get a lot of protein by putting together their everyday diet with respect to plant foods, for example, lentils, beans, chickpeas, tofu, tempeh, grains, nuts, seeds, and vegetables.

It is a typical mistake thinking that vegans do not get enough protein. The real issue is that most of the meat-eaters take in a lot of protein, which is connected to an assortment of infections! In case you are into wellness and expanding quality, you can add vegan protein powders to your diet for comfort, even though it is not vital.

Minerals

"There are a few minerals that are essential nutrients that people need to eat to be healthy. Minerals are synthetic components and cannot be integrated by any animal. All minerals are at last gotten from the earth, and the substance of minerals in plants shifts subject to the dirt they are developed in. Iron, zinc, and calcium are important minerals that people need to guarantee they acquire satisfactory measures." From *Human Herbivore*

Calcium – The best plant sources include kale, verdant Asian vegetables (like bok choy), rocket, calcium-set tofu, strengthened plant milk. (Check the mark and search for plant drains that have at any rate 120 mg calcium for every 100 ml.) Other plant foods that contain moderate measures of absorbable calcium are white beans, almonds, figs, and oranges.

Iron – great sources include vegetables, (for example, chickpeas, lentils, naval force beans, pinto beans, kidney beans, soybeans) tofu, tempeh, whole grains, braced vegan meat analogs, breakfast oats, pepitas, and green vegetables.

NOTE: *Vitamin-C rich foods (like squeezed orange, tomatoes, capsicum, and crude green vegetables) help to build the measure of iron we assimilate, so have a go at eating these foods in a similar meal. Tea and espresso can meddle with iron absorption, so it's best to have these between meals instead of with them.*

Zinc – sources include soy items, vegetables, nuts, seeds, whole grains, pepitas, and green vegetables.

Vitamins

Vitamins are essential nutrients that people need to get to be healthy. The main vitamins that are not easily obtained from natural plant foods are Vitamin B12 and Vitamin D. The various essential vitamins are promptly possible from eating a scope of plant foods, including vegetables, organic products, vegetables, nuts, seeds, and whole grains. It is important for anybody eating a plant-based diet to think about vitamin B12 and vitamin D and where to get them.

Vitamin D – the Sun! 10-30 minutes of day-by-day, gentle sun exposure, without sunscreen, is prescribed. During winter or for those living in less radiant zones, Vitamin D supplements are suggested.

Vitamin B12 – B12 is created by microscopic organisms and is found in fruit and minerals yet is rare in plant foods. (Eating fruit and minerals or unwashed vegetables is risky, so not prescribed!) People on plant-based diets can acquire vitaminB12 by eating sustained foods (for example, foods that have had vitamin B12 included, for example, a few soy milks, Marmite, and some meat analogs – check the mark. At any rate, three serves of vitamin B12-invigorated foods are required to meet the base prescribed intake.

The less demanding and the most solid approach to guarantee that you get satisfactory vitamin B12 is to take a vitamin B12 supplement. This can be either as an everyday multivitamin or vitamin B12 tablet, capsule, or fluid containing at any rate 100 mcg of vitamin B12 or a twice-week by week portion of 2000 mcg of vitamin B12. Women of regenerative age, newborn children, and kids must acquire enough vitamin B12 every day as it is essential for mental health and development.

Essential Fatty Acids

Essential unsaturated fats are parts of fats that people need to have in their diets. The two types of essential unsaturated fats that are required are called omega 6 unsaturated fats (of which linoleic acid is essential) and omega 3 unsaturated fats (of which alpha-linolenic acid is essential).

Omega 6 – linoleic acid is generally accessible from a scope of foods, including nuts, seeds, avocado, grains, and vegetable oils. We do not require a lot of omega 6, so even low-fat diets can give sufficient measures of linoleic acid.

Omega 3 – alpha-linolenic acid (ALA) is gotten from flaxseeds (sprinkle 2-3 tsps ground seeds over grain/muesli or add to a smoothie), chia seeds (make your own pudding) or flaxseed oil (shower over servings of mixed greens).

Our bodies need to change over the omega 3 ALA (from flaxseeds and so forth) to DHA and EPA, and we do this with variable proficiency. Another alternative to guarantee we get enough of this omega 3s is to supplement with algal-derived DHA/EPA. (Seaweed is the first source of omega 3s for fish.)

Trace Elements

Trace elements are mineral components that are required in limited quantities in human nutrition. They are gotten from fruit and minerals, and the measure of a specific trace component in a portion of food will rely upon the dirt the food was developed in. Lamentably present day cultivating strategies will, in general, exhaust the dirt of trace components, bringing about low rates in the foods developed on that dirt.

Iodine – sources include seaweed (e.g., nori algae) and iodized salt. Kelp (Kombu algae) is likewise wealthy in iodine yet not suggested because it can give an excessive amount of iodine, which could bring about harming the thyroid organ. In the event that salt is utilized, utilize iodized salt, and eating seaweed a couple of times each week will likewise support iodine intake. Another option is supplementation: multivitamin tablets containing around 100-150 micrograms of iodine will help guarantee a satisfactory iodine consumption.

Selenium – Brazil nuts are a rich source of selenium. Only one Brazil nut a day will prevent lack. Then again, most multivitamin supplements contain selenium.

CHAPTER 8

HIGH PROTEIN VEGAN RECIPES FOR ATHLETES

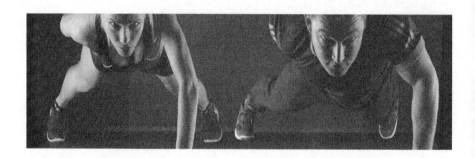

Going vegan in case you are an athlete is quite testing. Dynamic people need to get the perfect measure of protein, fats, and carbs. With an assortment of alternatives presently, it is considerably progressively advantageous to take in high protein food that you truly need to eat.

Vegan Breakfast Recipes

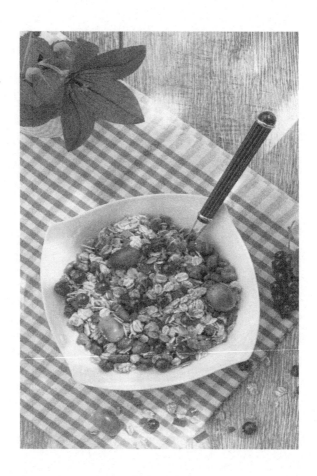

Vegan Breakfast Sandwich

Prep Time: 10 minutes

Cook Time: 10 minutes

Total Time: 20 minutes

Servings: three

Calories: 364kcal

Nutritional facts: 1sandwich, Calories: 365kcal, Carbohydrates: 51g, Protein: 16g, Fat: 12g, Saturated Fat: 5g, Sodium: 415mg, Potassium: 546mg, Fiber: 3g, Sugar: 6g, Vitamin A: 1280IU, Vitamin C: 8.4mg, Calcium: 137mg, Iron: 4.1mg

Ingredients:

- 1 tbsp of coconut oil

- 1 14 oz. tofu pack, pressed and cut longwise into 6 even cuts

- 1 tsp turmeric

- 1/two-tsp garlic powder

- 1/2 tsp Kala Nampak (dark salt)

- 3 vegan cheddar cuts

- 6 cuts of bread, or three wraps (sans gluten whenever preferred)

- 1-2 tbsp vegan mayo

- 1 cup of greens (spinach, spring blend, green lettuce, romaine, and so forth.)

- 1-2 medium tomatoes finely chopped

- 6 pickle cuts

- fresh split pepper, to taste

Preparation

1. Season one part of the tofu with salt, garlic powder, split pepper, and turmeric.

2. In a medium pan, heat oil over medium heat and put the tofu cuts seasoned side down on the pan. While the down side is cooking, season the upper side. Flip the cuts over and fry the other side for 3-5 minutes. Calculate the required time to pop the bread in the toaster whenever preferred.

3. To melt the vegan cheddar, on a baking paper, place 2 cuts of tofu one next to the other, with a cut of cheddar over each set. Put it on a grill pan for 1-3 minutes, until the cheddar is softened. You can likewise use the oven grill.

4. Spread mayo on the two sides of the bread. Put the two cuts of tofu with cheddar on one side. Add the greens and tomatoes (sprinkle with salt and pepper, whenever wanted). Finish it adding a few pickle cuts and close the sandwich together.

Notes: *Tofu - To begin, you should press the dampness out of the tofu. Put the tofu over a couple of paper towels and wrap it up. At that point, delicately press all the sides until the greater part of the dampness comes out. Do not over press. Cut the tofu down the middle and afterward cut every half into thirds, this will give both of you cuts for each sandwich.*

This recipe will make 3 breakfast sandwiches. If you might want to make less, you can store the leftover tofu in the refrigerator under water in a hermetically sealed holder for 3-4 days.

Kala Nampak (dark salt) is an Indian mineral salt that has a particular sulfurous smell and taste. It appears to escalate when heated up as well. This will include an 'eggy' smell and flavor to your tofu scramble recipe. I strongly suggest trying it in any event once. In case you are not into 'eggy' enhancement, you can utilize standard salt.

Vegan Crepes

Prep 5 m

Cool 2hrs

Cook 20 m

four servings

268 cals

Nutritional Facts: Per Serving: 268 calories; 12.1 g fat; 35.6 g starches; 4.3 g protein; 0 mg cholesterol; 295 mg sodium.

Ingredients:

- 1/2 cup soy milk

- 1/2 cup water

- 1/4 cup condensed soy margarine

- 1 tbsp turbinado sugar

- 2 tbsps maple syrup

- 1 cup wheat flour half whole

- 1/4 tsp salt

Preparation

1. In a large mixing bowl, blend the soymilk, water, 1/4 cup margarine, sugar, syrup, flour, and salt. Chill the batter for 2 hours.

2. Lightly oil a 5 to 6 inch skillet with some soy margarine. Warmth the skillet until hot. Then void around 3 batter tbsps into the skillet. Whirl to make the batter spread all over the skillet's base. Cook until browned, flip, and cook on the other side.

Mango Craze Juice Blend

Prep Time: 5 min

4 servings

150 cals

Nutritional Facts: Per Serving: 150 calories; 0.6 g fat; 38.4 g carbohydrates;1.3 g protein; 0 mg cholesterol; 9 mg sodium.

Ingredients:

- 3 cups diced mango

- 1/2 cups peach compote

- 1/4 cup orange flesh

- 1/4 cup pitted nectarine

- 1/2 cup pressed orange

- 2 cups ice

Preparation

1. Place mango, peaches, orange, nectarine, pressed orange, and ice into a blender. Blend for 1 minute, or until smooth.

Strawberry Oatmeal Smoothie

Prep Time: 5 mins

Servings: 2

Calories: 236 cals

Nutritional Facts: Per Serving: 235 calories; 3.7 g fat; 44.9 g carbohydrates; 7.6 g protein; 0 mg cholesterol; 65 mg sodium.

Ingredients:

- 1 cup of soymilk

- 1/2 cup moved oats

- 1 cut banana

- 14 fresh strawberries

- 1/2 tsp vanilla concentrate

- 1/2 tsps brown sugar

Preparation

1. In a blender, put soymilk, oats, banana, and strawberries. add vanilla and sugar at whatever point needed. Blend until smooth. Fill glasses and serve.

Country Style Fried Potatoes

Prep Time: 10 min

Cook Time: 15 min

Total Time: 25 min

Servings: 6

Calories: 326 cals

Nutritional Facts: Per Serving: 326 calories; 11.7 g fat; 52.1 g sugars; 4.8 g protein; 0 mg cholesterol; 400 mg sodium.

Ingredients:

- 1/3 cup shortening

- 6 big potatoes, peeled and cubed

- 1 tsp salt

- 1/2 tsp ground milled pepper

- 1/2 tsp garlic powder

- 1/2 tsp paprika

Preparation

1. in a large cast-iron skillet, heat shortening over medium-high warmth. Add potatoes and cook, occasionally

blending, until potatoes are perfectly bronzed. Season it with salt, pepper, the garlic powder, and the paprika. Serve hot.

Kale and Banana Smoothie

Prep Time: 5 min

Servings: 1

Calories: 311

Nutritional Facts: Per Serving: 312 calories; 7.3 g fat; 56.5 g carbohydrates;12.2 g protein; 0 mg cholesterol; 110 mg sodium.

Ingredients:

- 1 banana

- 2 cups cut kale

- 1/2 cup light unsweetened soy milk

- 1 tbsp flax seeds

- 1 tsp maple syrup

Preparation

1. Place the banana, kale, soy milk, flax seeds, and maple syrup into a blender. Blend until smooth. Serve over ice.

Homemade Soy Yogurt

Prep Time: 25 minutes

Calories: 141

Calories from Fat: 45

Nutritional Facts: Per Serving: Hard and fast Fat 5g; Drenched Fat 1g; Cholesterol 0mg; Sodium 36mg; Hard and fast Carbohydrates 14.3g; Dietary Fiber 1g; Sugars 9.6g; Protein 9g; vitamin A 0%; vitamin C 0%; Calcium1%; Iron 9%

Ingredients

- 3 tbsp cornstarch

- 1 32 oz. box unsweetened soymilk not chilled

- 1-2 tbsp date syrup

- 1 pack yogurt Starter

Preparation

1. put 2 cups of soymilk in a skillet and start warming by and by medium-low warmth. Be careful while warming since it can rise over the edge of the skillet or warm it too quickly.

2. Pour 1/2 cup of cold soymilk into a graduated container and add the 3 Cornstarch tbsps.

3. Once the milk in the pot starts to steam put in the cornstarch mix. Continue warming to and stir until it starts to thicken hardly.

4. Remove from the fire. Pour in the rest of the soymilk and let the temperature come down to at any rate 110 degrees F.

5. Whisk in the mixer to blend it.

Notes: *Presently you can make your own tasty soy yogurt easily in your kitchen. It thickens up magnificently. Include a little sweetness if you prefer or some fresh fruit after it is ready for a scrumptious choice for your breakfast.*

Pumpkin Pie Cake

Prep Time 20 minutes
Cook Time 25 minutes

Ingredients:

Wet Ingredients:

- 3/4 cup of pumpkin puree (or sweet potato puree)

- 1/4 cup of non-dairy milk

- 1 tsp vanilla

- 1/3 cup of maple syrup

- 2 tsp apple vinegar

- 1/4 cup sugar cane

Dry Ingredients:

- 1 cup wheat flour half whole

- 1/2 cup almond flour

- 1 Table pumpkin pie pizzazz

- 2 tsp baking powder

- 1/3 tsp sea salt

Preparation

1. Preheat the oven to 350°F (180C). Line an 8 x 8" heating dish with kitchen paper.

2. With a whisk, mix the whole of the wet fixings in a bowl.

3. Mix the dry ingredients in an ensuing bowl and add to the wet ones. Blend until just mixed.

4. Spread the batter uniformly into the heating dish.

5. Bake it for 30 minutes or until a toothpick or sharp cutting edge can stick in and come out dry. It may take a few minutes longer, depending upon your stove.

Note: *This sublimely great cake is not uncommon for fall but can be conveniently prepared in every period of the year with canned pumpkin or sweet potato puree.*

Vegan Lunch Recipes

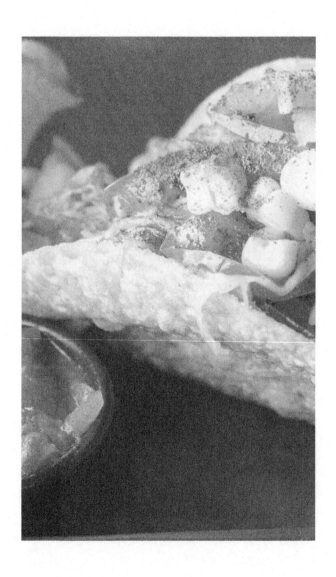

Crunchy Red Cabbage and Green Apple Sesame Slaw

Prep Time: 10 min

Serves 2

Ingredients:

For the plate of mixed greens:

- 3 cups gently chopped red cabbage

- 1 big granny smith apple crushed

- 2 tbsp. hemp seeds

For the dressing:

- 1/4 cup tahini

- 3 tbsps water

- 2 tsps agave nectar or maple syrup

- 1/2 tsp sesame oil

- 1/4 – 1/2 tsp sea salt (to taste)

- 1 tbsp squeezed apple vinegar

Preparation

1. Whisk dressing ingredients together and put them in a protected place.

2. Dress the chopped vegetables and hemp seeds with dressing; you can use as much as you want, yet be sure you dress everything properly (a half-cup will probably be enough). Slaw will keep in the refrigerator medium-term.

Plate of mixed greens

Prep Time: 10 min

Ingredients:

For the plate of mixed greens:

- 5 cups washed, dried, and hacked kale

- 2 little carrots, ground

- 2 stalk celery, hacked

- 4 tbsp. raisins

- 4 tbsp. hacked walnuts 1 apple, cut

For the dressing:

- 2 tbsp. olive oil

- 1/2 tbsp. squeezed apple

- 1 tbsp. agave

- Salt and pepper to taste

Preparation

1. Whisk the dressing ingredients together, and put them in a protected place .

2. In a large mixing bowl, pour about the dressing onto the hacked kale and start stirring it with your hands until the kale starts to get fully dressed. It should become even a little shriveled.

3. Add the rest of the plate of mixed greens, and prepare the whole serving of mixed greens again.

4. Plate the serving of mixed greens and top it with your cut apple. Enjoy. Scraps will keep medium-term in the cooler.

Smoky Avocado and Jicama Salad

Prep Time: 10 min

Serves: 2

Ingredients:

For the dressing:

- 1 small avocado

- 1 tbsp. cumin powder

- Juice of two limes

- 1/2 tsp smoked paprika

- 1 cup of water

- 1/4 tsp salt

- Cayenne pepper

For the serving of mixed greens:

- 1 cup crushed cabbage

- 1 cup crushed carrot

- 10 huge leaves romaine lettuce, roughly chopped

- 2 cups jicama, cut into matchsticks

- 2 tbsp. toasted pumpkin seeds

-

Preparation

1. Mix all dressing ingredients together in a blender until smooth.

2. Pour dressing over this plate of mixed greens, and mix. Serve.

Mango, Kale, and Avocado Salad

Prep Time: 10 min

Serves: 2

Ingredients:

- 1 pack wavy kale, chopped, washed, and dried (around 6 cups after preparation)

- Juice of 1 big lemon

- 2 tsps flax or olive oil

- 1-tsp sesame oil

- 2 tsps maple syrup or agave nectar

- Sea salt to taste

- 1 severed red ring pepper

- 1-cup mango, cut into little cubes

- 1 little Hass avocado, cut into cubes

Preparation

1. "Massage" the lemon juice, flax/olive and sesame oils, syrup, and salt into the kale until it has wilted and dressed consistently.

2. Blend in the pepper, mango, and avocado cubes. Serve.

Stewed Butternut Squash and Apple Soup

Prep Time: 15 min

Cook Time: 45 min

Total time: 1 hr

Servings: 4

Ingredients:

- 1 butternut squash, peeled and hacked (around 3-4 lbs., or 4-5 cups)

- 3 little apples, roughly hacked

- 1 next to no onion, hacked

- 2 tbsp. coconut oil

- 1/2 tsp real or sea salt (+more to taste)

- milled pepper to taste

- 1/4 tsp nutmeg

- One/2 tsp crushed thyme

- 2 1/2 cups low sodium vegetable soup

- 1/2 cup canned coconut milk

Preparation

1. Place squash, apples, and onion on a large cooking plate. Sprinkle coconut oil and salt and pepper over them, mix in with your hands, and meal at 375 degrees for around 45 minutes, or until they're all fragile and browned.

2. place cooked veggies in a blender with vegetable juices, nutmeg, coconut milk, and thyme. In case the soup needs more liquid, include some until it shows up the consistency you like.

3. Move soup to a pot, re-warmth, and serve.

Curried Yellow Lentils With Avocado

Prep Time:20 min
Cook Time:25 min
Total Time: 50 min
Serves: 4

Ingredients:

- 3/4 cup onion, diced

- 1/2 tbsp. coconut oil

- 1-cup yellow lentils

- 1 sweet potato, cut into 1/2 inch squares

- 2 carrots, diced

- 1/2 tsp turmeric

- 1 tbsp. yellow curry powder

- 1 tsp powdered ginger

- 1/2 tsp sea salt

- milled pepper to taste

- 4 cups vegetable squeeze or water

Preparation

1. Heat oil in a huge pot over medium warmth. Sauté onion until it is turning translucent and, to some degree, browned. Include the lentils, potato, carrots, and flavors/seasonings, and blend to solidify everything.

2. Add the soup or water to the pot and heat to the boiling point. Reduce to a stew and cook for 25 minutes, or until the lentils and sweet potato start melting.

3. Let lentils cool enough, then serve with fresh avocado cuts.

Kale Salad With Apple and Creamy Curry Dressing.

Prep Time: 15 min
Serving: 3-4

Ingredients:

For the dressing:

- 1/2 cup cashews or walnuts

- 2 tbsps lemon juice

- 2 pitted dates

- 1/2 cup water

- 1/2 tsp sea salt

- 2 tsp curry powder

For the plate of mixed greens:

- 1 head kale, washed, dried, and chopped (around 5 cups)

- 2 tremendous carrots, stripped and hacked

- 1 big apple, sliced into little pieces

- 1/3 cup raisins

- 1/2 cup chickpeas

Preparation

1. Mix all dressing fixings in a blender until smooth.

2. Massage the kale with the dressing, unti everything is wilted and dressed consistently. Add the apple, carrot, raisins, and chickpeas, and mix the plate of mixed greens, keeping all the additionally dressing in case you may want to add some more. Serve.

Red Quinoa, Cantaloupe, and Arugula Salad

Prep Time: 10 min

Servings: 2-3

Ingredients:

- 1/2 cup fresh melon, cut into cubes

- 1/2 cup red quinoa (classic quinoa is also totally fine)

- 4 cups arugula, stuffed

- 1/4 cup chopped, broken, or cut almonds

- 2 tbsps flax, hemp, or olive oil

- 1 tbsp squeezed apple vinegar

- 1-tsp maple syrup

- Sea salt and milled pepper to taste

Preparation

1. Whisk the oil together with vinegar, syrup, and seasoning.

2. Separate the arugula, quinoa, and melon onto two serving plates. Sprinkle them with almonds and a while later pour the dressing over.

Hot Thai Salad

Prep Time: 15 min

Serves 2

Ingredients:

For the dressing:

- 1 avocado

- 1 cup of coconut water

- ¼ cup cilantro

- ¼ cup basil

- ¼ tsp salt (or more)

- 2 pitted dates

- 1 tbsp. minced or ground ginger

- Sprinkle of cayenne pepper

For the plate of mixed greens:

- 1 ringer pepper, hacked

- 2 cups ground carrots

- 1/2 cup cilantro, hacked

- 1 cup grows

- 2 cups pulverized romaine lettuce

- 1 cup cut cucumbers

Preparation

1. Mix all dressing fixings in a quick blender until smooth.

2. Top the plate of mixed greens in with dressing as preferred. Serve.

Carrot Avocado Bisque

Prep Time: 10
Serves 2

Ingredients:

- 2 cups carrot juice

- 1/2 Hass avocado

- 1-tbsp low sodium tamari

- 1-tsp ground ginger

Preparation

1. Blend all fixings in a quick blender until smooth.

Gluten-free Tortilla Pizza

Prep Time: 20 min
Serves 2

Ingredients:

- 2 10" dull hued rice tortillas (Food for Life brand)

- 2/3 cup low sodium common marinara sauce

- 2 cups vegetable + garnishing of choice (broccoli, spinach, peppers, mushrooms, olives, artichokes, potato, etc.)

- 1/2 cup cashew cheddar

Preparation

1. Preheat the oven to 400 F. Place tortillas on a foil or cooking paper. Cook for 6/8 minutes, or until perceptibly firm.

2. Get tortillas out the oven. Top them up with tomato sauce and veggies, and put them back under the grill for 8/10 more minutes (until ingredients are cooked through). Sprinkle with cashew cheddar and serve.

Note: *If you do not have cashew cheddar, you can just sprinkle pizzas with dietary yeast. You can, as well , use red pepper hummus rather than the tomato sauce.*

Cashew Cheese

Prep Time: 10 min
Makes 1 cup

Ingredients:

- 1/4 cups cashews, soaked for at least three hours and drained

- 1/2 tsp sea salt

- 1 little clove garlic, minced (optional)

- 2 tbsp. lemon juice

- 1/3-1/2 cup water

- 1/4 cup healthy yeast

Preparation

1. Put the cashews, sea salt, garlic, lemon, and 1/3 cup water in a food processor. Blend them until the mix is extraordinarily smooth and soft (you are looking for a ricotta cheddar like surface), stopping to scratch the bowl down a few times and including some extra water when needed.

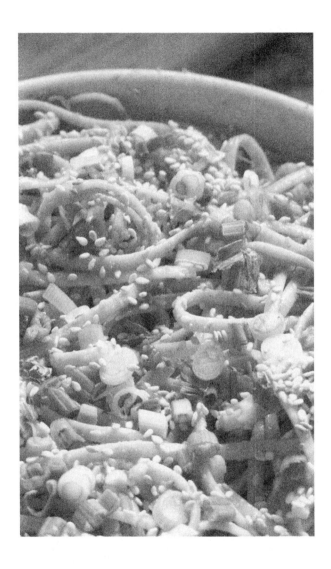

Beans and Quinoa Salad

Prep Time: 30 min

Serves: 4

Ingredients:

For the plate of mixed greens:

- 1-cup dry quinoa

- 2 cups vegetable soup or water

- 1/2 big cucumber, previously diced

- 1 little toll pepper, previously diced

- One can common dull beans

- 10-15 basil leaves, hacked into a chiffonade 1/4 cup fresh cilantro, sliced

for the vinaigrette:

- 2 tbsp. extra virgin olive oil

- 1/4 cup squeezed apple vinegar

- 1 tbsp. agave or maple syrup

- 1 tbsp. Dijon mustard

- 1 tsp cumin

- Salt and pepper to taste

Preparation

1. Wash quinoa in a strainer until the water runs clear. Move it to a little or medium pot and add two cups of vegetable stock or water and run of salt. Heat to the boiling point, then reduce it to a stew. Stew until quinoa has expended the total of the liquid and is delicate (around 15-20 minutes).

2. Move cooked quinoa to a mixing bowl. Add hacked vegetables, dim beans, and herbs.

3. Whisk dressing ingredients. Add the dressing to the plate of mixed greens, and serve. (If you do not feel that you need all the dressing, add less according to your preferences).

Note: *A plate of mixed greens is preserved for three days in the cooler.*

Zucchini Pasta, with Cherry Tomatoes, Basil, and Hemp Parmesan

Prep Time: 30 min
Serves: 4

Ingredients:

- Two big zucchini

- 1 red toll pepper, diced

- 15 cherry tomatoes, quartered

- Eight big basil leaves, chiffonade

- 2 small sweet potato, cut into cubes

- 2 tbsp. balsamic vinegar

- 1 small avocado, cubed

- 4 tbsp. hemp parmesan (recipe below)

Preparation

1. Utilize a spiralizer or a julienne peeler to cut zucchini into long strips.

2. Dress zucchini with all the ingredients, and serve.

Hemp Parmesan

Prep Time: 10 min

Makes 2/3 cup

Ingredients:

- 6 tbsp. hemp seeds

- 6 tbsp. dietary yeast

- Sea salt

Preparation

Unite all ingredients in a food processor, and wihsk them until uniform. Store in the cooler for whatever up to fourteen days.

Gluten-free White Bean and Summer Vegetable Pasta

Prep Time: 30 min
Serves: 4

Ingredients:

- 1 little eggplant, cut into approx 1 inch cubes and slightly salted for 30 minutes, then squeezed dry

- 1 clove garlic, minced

- 1 big zucchini, cut

- 1 or 2 diced tomatoes

- 1 little can common tomato sauce

- 1 tsp agave

- 1 tbsp. dried basil

- 1 tsp dried oregano

- 1 tsp dried thyme

- 1 can (or 2 cups previously cooked) cannellini

- 8 oz. dry dim shaded rice or quinoa pasta (rigatoni, linguine, and penne are all in all fine)

Preparation

1. Heat a large skillet with some olive or coconut oil (or use two or three tbsp. water).

2. Include the zucchini and cook it until needed

3. Include the canned tomatoes, tomato sauce, agave, basil, oregano, thyme. Heat through. Taste it and add a measure of whatever herbs you like.

4. Add the white beans and heat the whole sauce through. This is so scrumptious, you could eat it by itself as a "cheater's" ratatouille.

5. While the sauce is cooking, put a pot of salted water to boil. Put in pasta when fully boiling, and cook it until needed, preferably still to a little hard (al dente).

6. Drain the pasta, cover with sauce and serve.

Note: *Leftovers can be stored for three days in the cooler.*

Butternut Squash Curry

Prep Time: 40-45 min

Serves: 4

Ingredients:

- 1 tbsp coconut oil

- 1 white or yellow onion, hacked

- 1 clove garlic, minced

- 1 tbsp new ginger, minced

- 3 tbsps red curry stick

- 1-tbsp sugar cane or coconut sugar

- 2/3 cups vegetable soup

- One 14- 15 oz coconut

- 1-tbsp soy sauce or tamari

- 1 green or red toll pepper, cut

- 1 pound butternut squash

- 1 to 2 tbsp lime juice

Preparation

1. Heat the coconut oil in an enormous pot or wok. Add the onion and cook until it is wilted and slightly browned (5 to 8 minutes).

2. Add the garlic and the ginger and let them cook for about a minute. Then, add the curry paste and sugar. Add the ingredients until the paste is uniform.

3. Put in the stock, the coconut milk, and the tamari. Add the red pepper and butternut squash. Stew until the squash is completely melted (25 to 30 minutes).

4. Mix in the green beans and let them cook for a couple of minutes, or until fragile. Season the curry to taste with extra soy sauce or tamari and blend in the lime press as needed. Remove from heat and serve over quinoa or dark basmati rice.

Note: *Remains can be stored 4 days in the cooler.*

Zucchini Alfredo with Basil and Cherry Tomatoes

Prep Time: 20 min

Serves: 2

Ingredients:

- 2 big zucchini

- 1-cup cherry tomatoes split

- 1/4 cup basil, cut

- Rough vegan Alfredo sauce

- 1-cup cashews, soaked for at least three hours and drained

- 1/3 cup water

- 1 tbsp agave or maple syrup

- 1 clove garlic

- 3-4 tbsp. lemon juice

- 1/4 cup healthy yeast

- 1/4 tsp sea salt

Preparation

1. Use a julienne peeler or a spiralizer to cut zucchini into long strips (looking like noodles).

2. Add tomatoes and basil to the zucchini noodles

3. Blend all of the Alfredo sauce ingredients together in a blender until smooth.

4. Cover the pasta in 1/2 cup sauce, and mix it in well, add the remaining sauce. Serve.

Vegan Dips and Dressings

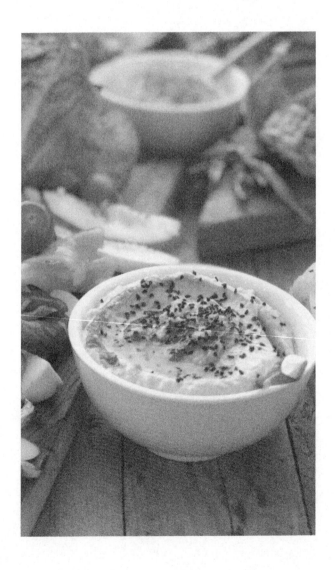

Turmeric Tahini Dressing

Prep Time: 5 min
Serves: ½

Ingredients:

- 1/2 cup tahini

- Two tbsps squeezed apple vinegar

- 2 tbsps of the coconut aminos or tamari

- 1/2 tsp of ground ginger (or 1 tsp new, ground ginger)

- 2 tsps turmeric

- 1 tsp maple syrup

- 2/3 - 3/4 cup water

Preparation

Combine all ingredients in a blender or food processor until smooth. Start with 2/3 cup water and add more when needed.

Walnut Pesto

Prep Time: 10 min
Serves: 1 generous cup

Ingredients:

- 1 cup coarsely severed walnuts

- 2 1/2 cups stuffed fresh basil leaves, washed and dried

- 1 big garlic clove

- 1 tbsp. lemon finds a good pace

- Juice of one lemon

- 1/4 cup healthful yeast

- 1/2 cup great extra virgin olive oil

- Salt and pepper to taste

Preparation

1. Granulate walnuts in a food processor until finely ground. Add basil and beat until it shapes a coarse mix.

2. Add the garlic, lemon juice, and dietary yeast, and beat for two or three more minutes. Add olive oil in a thin stream.

Balsamic Tahini Dressing

Prep Time: 10 min
Serves: 1 cup

Ingredients:

- 1/2 cup of tahini

- 1/4 cup of balsamic vinegar

- 1/2 cup of water.

- 1/4 tsp of the garlic powder, or 1/2 clove finely minced garlic

- 1 tbsp. of tamari or name shouts

- ½ tsp dried oregano

- 1 clove garlic

- 3 tbsp. fresh dill

- 3 tbsp. fresh parsley

- 3 tbsp. olive oil

Preparation

1. Blend all ingredients in a blender and serve.

Rich Apricot Ginger Dressing

Prep Time: 30 min
Serves: about 2 cups

Ingredients:

- 1/2 cup dried apricots, pressed

- 3/4 inch long handles unrefined ginger (or 1/2 tsp ginger powder)

- 1/2 cup pressed orange

- 1/2 cup water

- 2 tbsp. squeezed apple vinegar

- 1 lbsp. tamari

- 2 tbsp. olive oil

Preparation

1. Put all dressing ingredients in a blender, blend and serve.

Fig and White Balsamic Vinaigrette

Prep Time: 30 min
Serves: ½ cup

Ingredients:

- 6 big dried figs soaked for about 8 hours

- 1/3 white balsamic vinegar

- 1/4 cup olive oil

- 1/4 water

- 1 little clove garlic

- 1 tbsp. Dijon mustard

- Salt and dim pepper to taste

Preparation:

1. Blend all ingredients in a blender till completely smooth. Add more water if the result is too thick.

Vegan Snacks

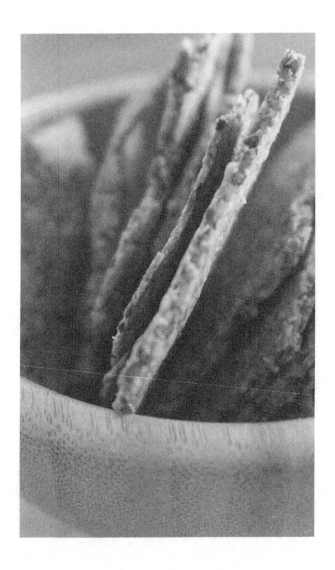

Vegan Peanut Butter

Prep Time: 30 min

Serves: about 2 cups

Calories: 218

Nutrition Facts: Sugar: 15.6g; Sodium: 55mg; Fat: 14.6g; Saturated Fat: 6.5g; Carbohydrates: 19.2g; Fiber: 1.7g; Protein: 4.1g

Ingredients:

- 1 cup (250g) Smooth Creamy Peanut Butter

- 1/3 cup (80ml) Vegan Whipped Cream

- 2 cups (240g) Icing Sugar

- 10.5oz (300g) Vegan Chocolate

- 1 tsp Coconut Oil

  For Decoration (Optional):

- Crushed Peanuts

Preparation

1. Add the nutty spread and powdered sugar to the mixing bowl and with the electric blender on low-speed mix it in. It will be weak.

2. Slowly stir in the vegan whipped cream until getting a thick consistency that you can easily shape into small balls. You may not need to add all the whipped cream, it depends upon the kind of peanut butter you're using, take care to stir in the whipped cream little by little.

3. When your peanut butter mix is ready, cover a plate with kitchen paper, shape the spread mix into small balls and place the plate into the cooler for a couple of hours until the balls have set distinctly.

4. Break up the vegan chocolate and place it into a microwave-safe dish. Microwave in 30-second repeatedly, taking it out to blend at evenly spaced times. Add the coconut oil and blend it in (makes the chocolate increasingly thin and less challenging to work with).

5. Place each ball in the mellowed chocolate and use two tsps to cover it in chocolate and a little later lift it out and

place it back onto the paper lined plate. Sprinkle with crushed peanuts (optional).

6. When all the balls are covered in chocolate, place in the cooler for around 10 minutes for the chocolate to set.

7. Keep the balls stored in the refrigerator and serve directly from the cooler.

Hemp Hummus

Prep Time: 15 min
Serves: 4

Ingredients:

- 1/4 cup shelled hemp seeds

- 1 can chickpeas, drained, or two cups normally cooked chickpeas

- 1/2 tsp salt (to taste)

- 2-3 tbsp. normally squashed lemon juice (to taste)

- 1 little clove garlic, minced

- 1 tbsp. tahini (optional)

- 1/2 tsp cumin

Preparation

1. Place the hemp seeds in the bowl of a food processor and squash them well.

2. Add the chickpeas, salt, lemon, garlic, tahini, and cumin, and begin to mix. Add water for a thin stream (stopping to scratch the bowl multiple times) until the mix is perfectly smooth.

3. Topping with extra hemp seeds and serve. Hummus will keep in the cooler for up to four days.

Peanut Butter And Jelly Snack Balls

Prep Time: 30 min

Serves: 20 balls

Ingredients:

- 1/2 cups unsalted peanuts

- 1/2 cups dull raisins

- 2 tbsps nutty spread

- Pinch of sea salt

Preparation

1. Add all ingredients to a food processor and work them until the mix is starting to stay together. It may release a little oil, yet that is OK.

2. Shape the mix into 1-inch balls. Store in the cooler for any occasion, pull out thirty minutes before serving.

Sweet Potato Hummus

Prep Time: 30 min
Serves: 6
Calories: 218
Nutrition Facts: Sugar: 15.6g; Sodium: 55mg; Fat: 14.6g; Saturated Fat: 6.5g; Carbohydrates: 19.2g; Fiber: 1.7g; Protein: 4.1g

Ingredients:

- 2 cups sweet potato, steamed or prepared and cut into cubes

- 1 can dried chickpeas (or 1/2 cups cooked chickpeas)

- 1/2 tsp sesame oil

- 1/4 cup tahini

- 1 tbsp lemon juice

- 1/2 tsp smoked paprika

- 1/2 tsp salt

- Milled pepper to taste

- 1/2 cup water

Preparation

1. Place sweet potato, chickpeas, sesame oil, tahini, lemon, salt, and pepper into a food processor. Beat to mix.

2. Start the blender and pour in the water. Mix it all, stopping a few times to scratch down the bowl. Add more water until you have a rich, smooth, completed hummus. Serve.

Vegan Za'atar Crackers

Prep Time: 10 min
Cook Time: 15 min
Total Time: 25 min
Calories: 826kcal
Nutrition Facts: Carbohydrates: 167g; Protein: 21g; Fat: 6g; Sodium: 1177mg; Potassium: 425mg; Fiber: 7g; Sugar: 5g; Vitamin A: 150IU; Vitamin C: 2mg; Calcium: 195mg; Iron: 14.6mg

Ingredients:

- ⅔ cup flour

- ½ tsp baking powder

- 1/two tsp salt

- 1 tsp of olive oil.

- 1/2 cup water

- 1 tsp maple syrup

Preparation

1. Preheat the stove to 400°F (200°C)

2. In a mixing bowl put the flour, baking powder, and salt. Whisk, and a little later add olive oil and water. Mix in with a wooden spoon until it gets together. Check with your hand until it is a smooth blend. Add more flour if the batter needs it.

3. On a gently floured kitchen paper, spread the batter as thin and even as possible. Use more flour in case you need to.

4. Blend 1 tbsp of water in with 1 tsp of maple syrup and brush the top of the wafers with this mix. Then, sprinkle the za'atar seasoning on top.

5. Cut it with a pizza shaper length and widthwise into separated wafers.

6. Heat them in the oven for around 15 minutes until they get crisp and darker. Let them cool a little before diving in. They are delectable with your favourite kind of hummus.

Note: *to store, let them chill completely, by then put them in a cookie box thusly, they will stay firm and luscious!*

Vegan Smoothies

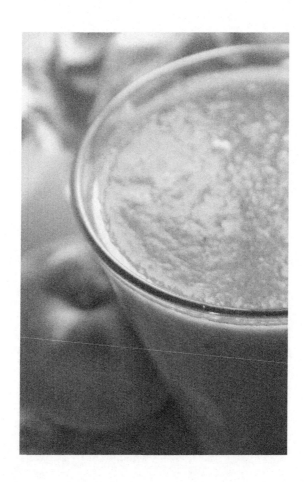

Avocado Banana Nuts Smoothie

Prep Time: 10 min
Serves:1
Calories: 806
Nutritional Facts: Per Serving: 57.2 g fat; 66.8 g starches;
18.8 g protein; 0 mg cholesterol; 401 mg sodium.

Ingredients:

- 1 cup almond milk

- 1 avocado, peeled and pitted

- 1 big banana, cut into pieces

- 3 tbsps smooth nutty spread

- 2 ice cubes

- 1 tsp vanilla concentrate (optional)

Preparation

1. Mix almond milk, avocado, banana, nutty spread, ice cubes, and vanilla in a blender until smooth.

Banana Hemp Seed Smoothie

Prep Time: 10 min
Serves:1
Calories: 250
Nutritional Facts: Per Serving:; 12 g fat; 34.9 carbs; 5.4 g protein; 0 mg cholesterol; 83 mg sodium.

Ingredients:

- 10 min., two servings, 250 cals

- 2 bananas

- 1 cup fresh peach cuts

- 2 tbsps almond spread

- 1 tbsp hemp seeds

- 2 cups of water

Preparation

1. Layer bananas, peach cuts, almond spread, and hemp seeds in a blender; pour in water. Spread and blend until smooth.

Mango Tahini Smoothie

Prep Time: 10 min
Serves:1
Calories: 200 cal
Nutritional Facts: Per Serving:; 9.6 g fat; 32.5 g carbs; 3.5 g protein; 0 mg cholesterol; 24 mg sodium.

Ingredients:

- 10 min., two servings, 200 cals

- 2 cups fresh mango cut

- 1 cup of water

- 2 tbsps tahini

- 2 tbsps lime juice

Preparation

1. Mix mango, water, tahini, and lime press together in a blender until smooth.

Cucumber Pear Smoothie

Prep Time: 10 min
Serves:1
Calories: 165 cal
Nutritional Facts: Per Serving:; 0.5 g fat; 42 carbs; 3.9 g protein; 0 mg cholesterol; 11 mg sodium.

Ingredients:

- 1/4 cucumber, cut

- 1 pear, cut

- 1/4 cup fresh pineapple

- 2 tbsps canned white beans

- 1 tbsp cut fresh parsley

- 1/2 tsp ground fresh ginger

- 1/2 cup water, or as needed

Preparation

1. Layer cucumber, pear, pineapple, white beans, parsley, and ginger in a blender, including water. Spread and blend the mix until smooth, including more water for a more fluid smoothie.

Smoothie Bowl with Mango and Coconut

Prep Time: 10 min
Serves:1
Calories: 442
Nutritional Facts: Per Serving:; 10.6 g fat; 90.3 carbs; 4.4 g protein; 0 mg cholesterol; 180mg sodium.

Ingredients:

- 1/2 cups fresh mango pieces

- 1 cup vanilla-prepared almond milk

- 1 fresh banana

- 1 tbsp unsweetened coconut cream

- 1/four-tsp vanilla concentrate

- 1 tbsp slashed coconut

- 1 tsp goji berries

- 1/two tsp chia seeds

Preparation

1. Place mango pieces, almond milk, banana, coconut cream. and vanilla in a blender; puree until thick and smooth. Fill a serving bowl.

2. Top smoothie bowl with chipped coconut, goji berries, and chia seeds.

Notes: *You can use any vanilla-prepared milk. Use less milk in case you favor a thicker smoothie.*

Cashew Butter Smoothie with Banana, Berry, Dates, and Flax

Prep Time: 10 min
Serves:1
Calories: 400
Nutritional Facts: Per Serving:; 17g fat; 59.9 carbs; 8.4 g protein; 0 mg cholesterol; 90 mg sodium.

Ingredients:

- 5 min., 1 serving, 400 cals

- 1 big banana

- 1/2 cup cold unsweetened almond milk

- 1/3 cup fresh blueberries

- 2 dates pitted

- 1/2 tbsps flax seeds

- 1 tbsp cashew butter

Preparation

1. Mix a banana, almond milk, blueberries, dates, flax seeds, and cashew margarine together in a blender on quick until smooth.

Printed in Great Britain
by Amazon

36006781R00136